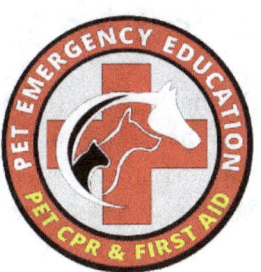

Published by

Professional Credits

We would like to dedicate this book to all the animal lovers out there who believe that every animal deserves a chance.

Printed by Pet Emergency Education, LLC Las Vegas, NV USA

Preface

Pet Emergency Education, LLC makes every reasonable attempt to provide high-quality, up-to-date and accurate information at the time of publication. Emergency education is in no way a substitute for professional veterinary medical care, diagnosis, and treatment.

The authors, reviewers, editors, and publisher have made extensive efforts to ensure that the information contained in this book is accurate and conforms to the standards accepted at the date of publication. The reader is advised to discuss information obtained in this book with a veterinarian or other qualified animal health practitioner.

In a study conducted by veterinary emergency organizations, it was discovered that improving the variations in CPR technique as performed on dogs and cats would improve the survival rates for cardiopulmonary resuscitation.

Our programs are based on the most current veterinary industry-standard methods of animal emergency first aid. These methods were developed by veterinarians and have been researched and validated. It has been shown that one out of four pets would survive a medical emergency if just one first aid technique is administered prior to receiving veterinary care. The method of CPR that we teach has been researched and proven to increase survival rates in animals experiencing cardiopulmonary arrest.

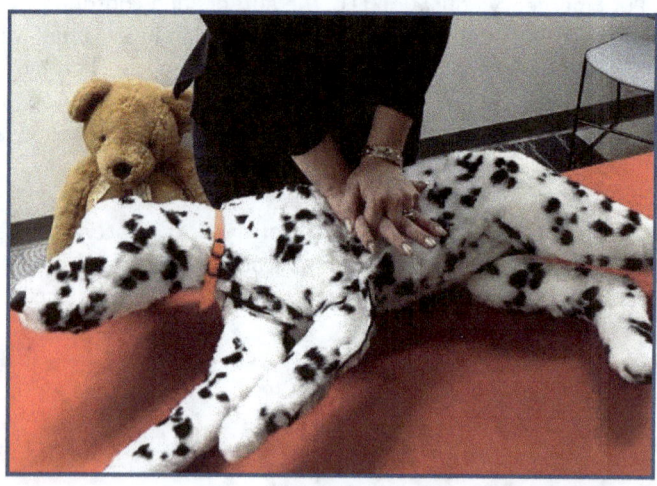

About Us

Pet Emergency Education is a family owned and operated company that strives to provide the highest quality animal CPR, first aid and emergency response training to veterinary and animal professionals, pet owners, emergency responders and anyone else who genuinely cares for animals. Our internationally recognized programs offer detailed, hands-on training providing participants with a well-rounded education.

Our programs are recognized by local and national veterinary associations, the American Association of Veterinary State Boards, the Certification Council for Professional Dog Trainers, Pet Sitters International and International Association of Animal Behavior Consultants, among others. We've partnered with hundreds of reputable animal related businesses and we are proud to generously give back to the community through our shelter/rescue fundraiser programs.

Our programs are based on researched and proven successful methods of animal CPR developed by emergency veterinarians and are among the most recognized Pet CPR certifications in the US and Canada. Instructors are veterinary and animal professionals with experience in emergency management and who are certified by the Federal Emergency Management Agency in Animal Disaster Preparedness and Emergency Response. Our certification is recognized by employers, veterinary organizations, shelters, rescues, disaster response teams and more. Pet Emergency Education is unlike any other animal emergency certification company; we were founded by a Credentialed Veterinary Technician with 25+ years of experience working in veterinary hospitals, who also has taught veterinary emergency and critical care in higher education and is the author of four textbooks. The founder is also certified in Basic and Advanced Life Support by the American College of Emergency and Critical Care and Cornell University.

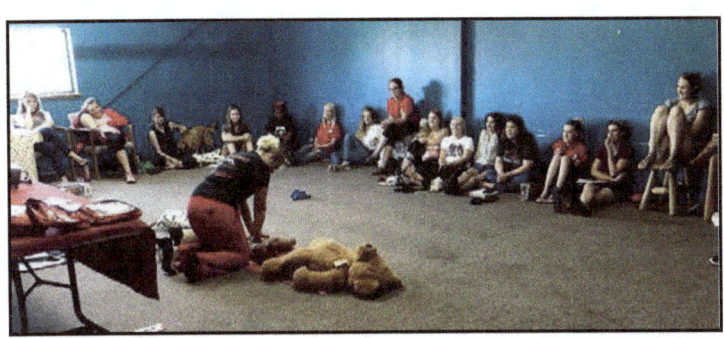

Introduction

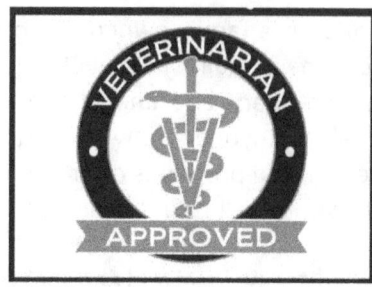

"According to the American Animal Hospital Association (AAHA), 1-out-of- 4 more pets would survive a medical emergency if just one first aid technique were applied prior to receiving veterinary care."

Pet first aid is the Immediate help that is given to an injured or ill pet until professional help is available.

This training in no way should replace veterinary care, however, it may increase your pet's chance of survival and/or lessen the severity of a pet's condition. Rapid recovery of a beloved animal relieves stress on your family and your pet, it can save you a considerable amount of money for veterinary care, and most importantly, when you're trained in first aid and CPR you may be able to save a precious life!

This book not only covers CPR and first aid, but it also outlines some basic health information for dogs and cats that may need the attention of a veterinarian.

As stated by the American Veterinary Medical Association, first aid administered to an animal should always be followed by immediate veterinary care. Although first aid care is not a substitute for veterinary care, it can save an animal's life until it receives veterinary treatment.

This book does not replace professional pet first aid training and it is strongly suggested that anyone reading this text obtains proper training before managing an emergency with a pet.

Be Prepared- The Importance of the Pet First Aid Kit

Medical emergencies that involve animals should have first aid administered immediately. These situations are considered a health crisis and many can become life threatening very quickly. Appropriate first aid measures can keep your animal alive until you are able to get to a veterinary hospital, can prevent a traumatic injury from getting worse and alleviate pain for your pet. Any pet owner, animal lover and animal business professional needs to have the essential first aid supplies handy if and when an emergency occurs with an animal. A first aid kit for dogs, cats, horses and people is a vital component in an emergency disaster preparedness plan as well. Pet Emergency Education sells veterinary-approved pet first aid kits on our website at www.petemergencyeducation.com. Details about the kits can be seen on the next page. It is suggested that you have at least one full-size first aid kit in your home or animal business plus one travel-size kit in your car, backpack, camping gear, etc.

First aid kits need to have a variety of medical supplies in them so that no matter what the emergency you have what you need to manage it. There are several commercial first aid kits available for purchase at retail stores and online websites focused on animal care however we strongly recommend the Pet Emergency Education Deluxe Pet First Aid Kit. Make sure to be knowledgeable about what supplies you need so you can find a kit that best suits you and your pet. People sometimes choose to build their own kit, but if you weigh the cost it is likely the same price or cheaper to purchase a ready-made kit from a retailer. These retail kits often come in durable waterproof cases and include quite a few valuable items. If you intend to take your dog on a boat, fishing, camping, or anywhere that water may be a factor, having a waterproof first aid kit is an important consideration.

Recommended Emergency Documentation for the Pet

Be sure to have important phone numbers such as the animal's regular veterinarian, the nearest 24-hour emergency veterinary clinic, poison control, animal control, and friend and/or relative that can help you in an emergency situation. Have a copy of the pet's medical and vaccine records available. If you need to seek veterinary care at a clinic that is not the one you routinely take your animal to you likely will have to present current medical history to them to receive treatment for your pet. In a natural disaster, local shelters may also require up to date vaccines for an animal to stay there.

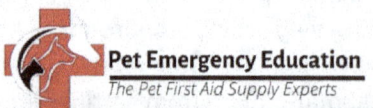
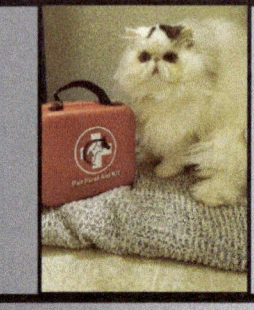
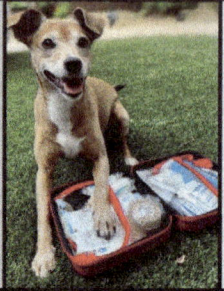
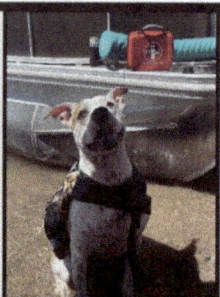
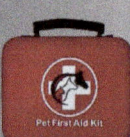

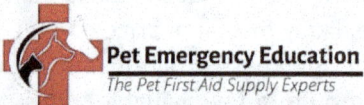
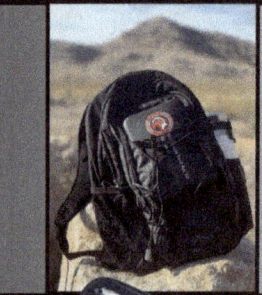
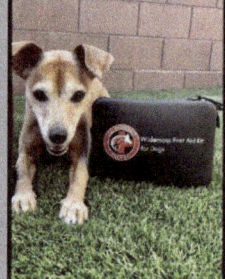
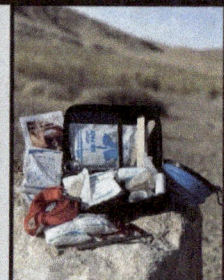
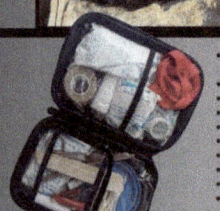

Your Own Safety

Dogs and cats are considered predatory species, meaning that they have strong instincts to prey on other lesser species. These instincts include aggressive behaviors by nature to catch and eat prey as well as to defend themselves. Although domestic dogs and cats have been "tamed" so to speak, they still have many of those instinctual defense mechanisms which, if faced with a life-threatening and/or painful situation, may cause them to lash out aggressively, potentially causing harm to their rescuer(s).

You need to know how to recognize aggressive signs in dogs and cats. These species have recognizable behaviors that one can identify before approaching the animal. Do not think that your own pet will never bite you. Even the cuddliest, fuzziest, and sweetest animal can bite if it feels threatened.

The most important thing to remember when approaching an injured or ill animal is to *approach with caution*. When an animal is injured or ill it may be scared and in pain. Their first reaction from a predator is usually to scramble to get away, or to bite or scratch to protect itself.

Cats and dogs communicate through body language. When using body language to interpret the message an animal is trying to get across, it is important to consider both the context and the animal's individual personality. While certain physical cues commonly appear in both cats and dogs, those cues don't always mean the same things, and it's important to know the differences to better understand the cat or dog.

Here are a few examples of behaviors that may communicate dramatically different things between dogs and cats.

Tail held high:

When a cat holds its tail high, it can signal that they are friendly and relaxed. The higher the cat's tail, the more confident they may be. However, if their tail is raised high with the fur erect and puffed out, it usually indicates alarm or even be a sign of aggression. When a dog holds his tail high, on the other hand, it often signals high arousal and the possibility of aggressive behavior. A dog that is agitated may also flick their tail back and forth vigorously. A dog is more likely to carry his tail in a neutral position, extended out behind him, when they are relaxed.

Wagging tail:

Friendly dogs wag their tail loosely back and forth at medium height. When a cat's tail begins to wag back and forth, an unfriendly encounter might occur.

Closed mouth:

Relaxed cats have closed mouths; relaxed dogs may have a closed or partially open mouth. The more tense a dog is, the more tightly closed their mouth may become, although a very stressed dog may pant heavily or yawn.

Ears up for greeting:

A cat who is confident greeting people will normally hold their ears forward and alert. If their ears move backward or twitch, it may indicate uncertainty. By contrast, one sign of a friendly dog is that the dog's ears move back just slightly. A submissive dog will move their ears back even further as an appeasement gesture. Dogs with erectly pricked ears may be ready to stand their ground against another animal if necessary, however this behavior is specific to the individual dog.

Turning to the side:

Both dogs and cats turn their bodies to the side when attempting to shut off a potential threat. A dog may do this in order to show that he means no harm, while a cat may be trying to appear larger and more threatening to their opponent.

Lying belly up:

A dog is likely to lie on their back as a submissive greeting behavior or as a way to get their belly rubbed by someone. A cat, on the other hand, will lie on their back in self-defense; this position allows them to have all four paws, with claws drawn, ready to react to any threat. A cat will sometimes lie on their back for people they feel comfortable with however very few cats enjoy having their belly rubbed and may respond aggressively.

Other warning signs are growling, snarling, barking, pinning of the ears back, and tail swishing.

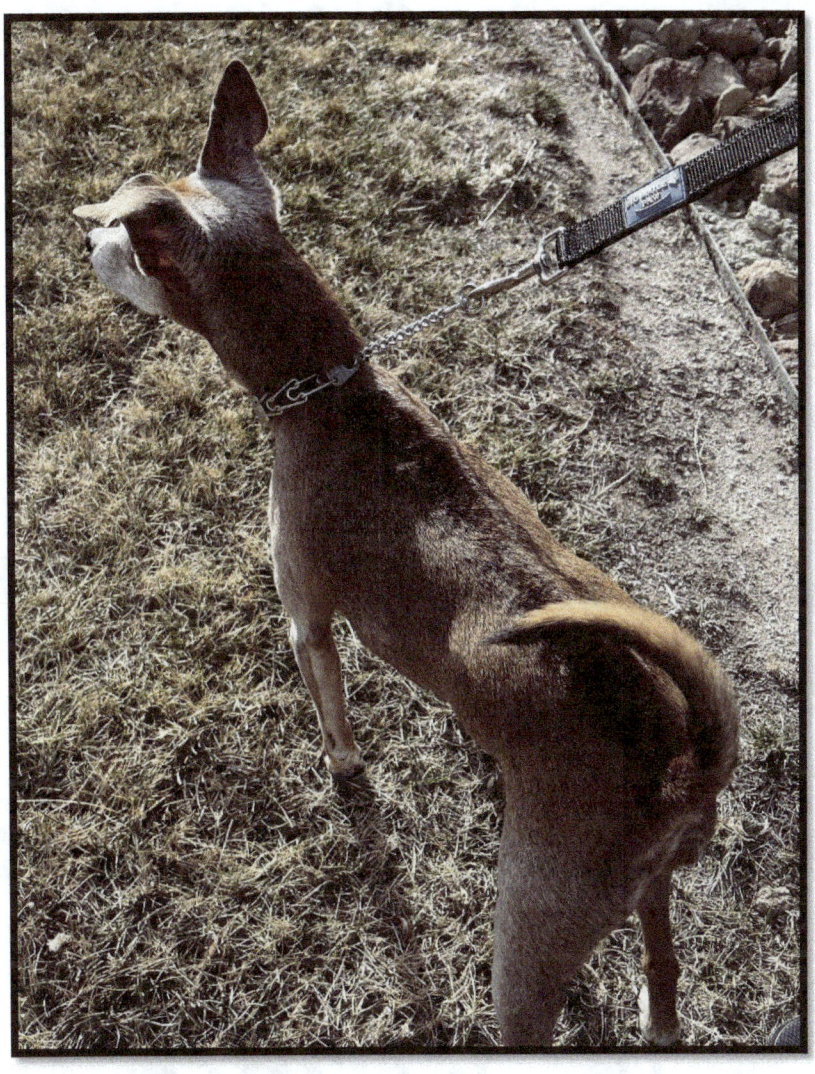

Note the hair standing up on this dog's neck and back. This is called Piloerection which is the erection or bristling of hairs due to the involuntary contraction of small muscles at the base of hair follicles that occurs as a reflexive response of the sympathetic nervous system especially to cold, shock, or fright.

How to Approach an Injured Animal

Approach the animals slowly and speak calmly to them. Observe their behavior as you get closer to determine if you will need to place a muzzle, blanket, or another restraint-assisting device on them. We will discuss moving and transporting an injured animal in the next section.

If you can get close enough to touch the animal, do so on its rear end. Remember, the front-end bites so you want to touch them as far from their mouth as possible to see how the animal will react. Even if the animal does not react to your touch, continue to work slowly and cautiously.

Cats are a bit more reactive than dogs. Cats also have the added means of defense, scratching. Having a blanket or towel handy is good when working with cats. You can use it to wrap the cat up so it cannot scratch you.

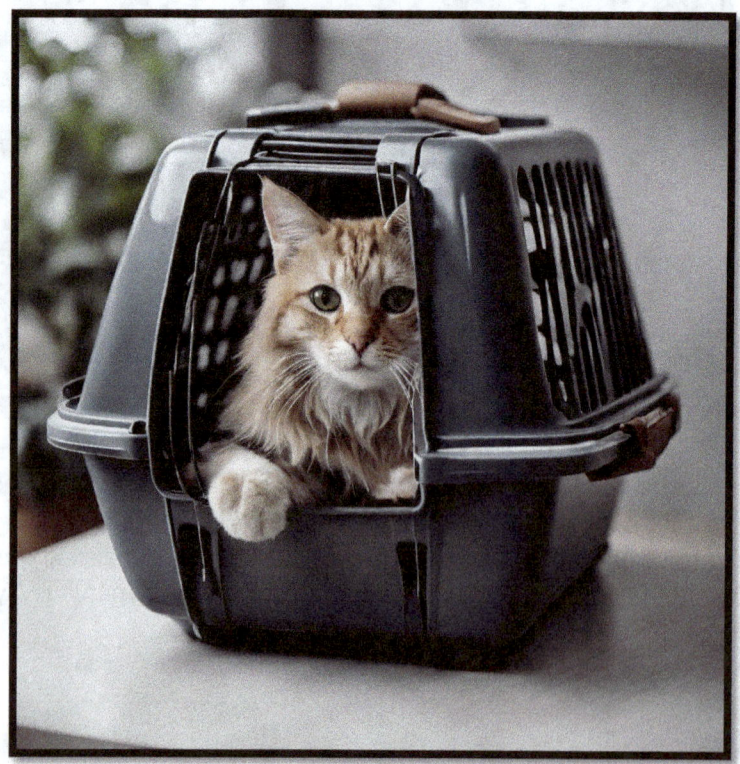

Transporting a cat in a carrier is a safe way to move them as long as they are not experiencing a life-threatening condition that needs to be tended to enroute to veterinary care

At the Scene of the Emergency

When you arrive at the location of an animal that is in trouble the first thing you should try to do if you are not the owner of this animal is to identify the owner. Although the laws in each state vary when it comes to legal liability, it is in the rescuer's best interests to find the owner and gain permission to provide aid to the animal. Check the Good Samaritan Laws in your state to understand the regulations that will apply to you.

Regulations Surrounding Pet CPR

Laws and regulations regarding both human and animal CPR vary by state. It is hard to say whether performing pet CPR is legal in most areas as the veterinary practice laws are very vague. In general, a person who is trained in first aid response for dogs and cats should freely be able to do so without concern. Veterinarians welcome pet owners to learn first aid and emergency response for their pets. It ensures the potential of a more positive outcome for the animal and many veterinary clinics host pet CPR classes for their clients. If you have questions about your state regulations, please contact your local veterinary medical board.

How to Transport a Sick and/or Injured Animal

Moving an animal can potentially do more harm than good. Some trauma injuries require minimal movement, or the condition can be worsened. Try to minimize movement of the head, neck, and spine and If possible, place the animal on a flat, hard surface like a piece of wood. Placing small animals in a box or crate can reduce stress and keep the animal, as well as yourself, as safe and comfortable as possible. A good rule of thumb is to move the animal as still as possible but support their body in a straight line from their nose to their tail.

For many animals that you can carry in your arms, place one arm under the shoulders and the other arm under its hips. Support their head on your elbow and hug their back into your stomach as you lift them. If it is a large dog that you cannot lift by yourself then you will need to enlist the help of a family member, friend, or neighbor to assist you. See the pictures on the next page on how to transport a pet.

Proper Way to Transport an Injured Animal

1. Position yourself behind the animal. It is best if the animal is lying on its right side.

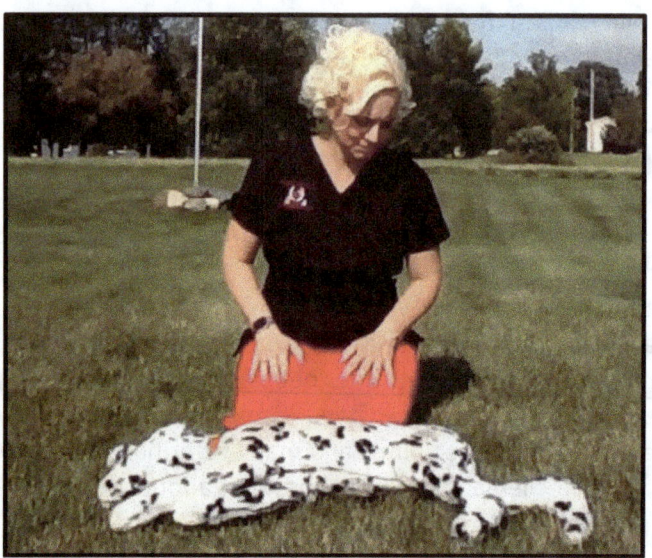

2. Place your forearm under the animal's hips as seen below.

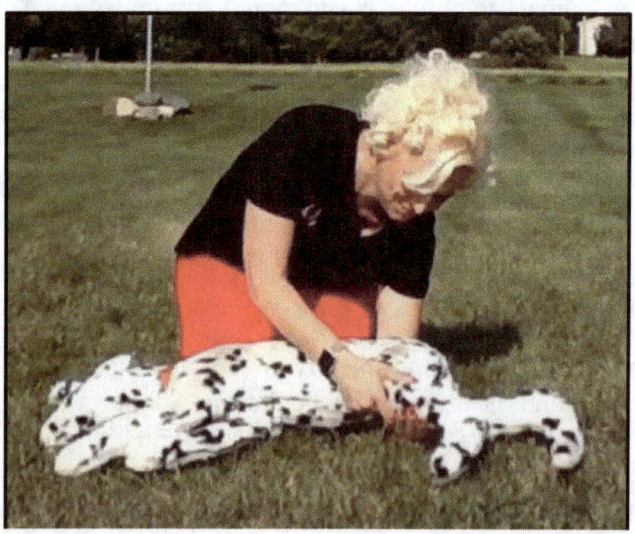

3. Place your other forearm under the animal's shoulders as pictured below.

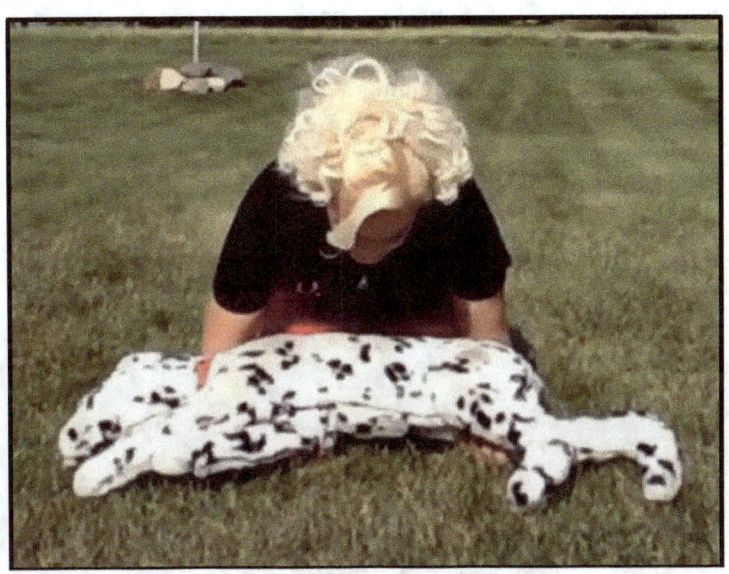

4. Finally brace the animal's back against your stomach and lift them carefully. Move as swift but as still as possible to move the animal without bouncing them around too much.

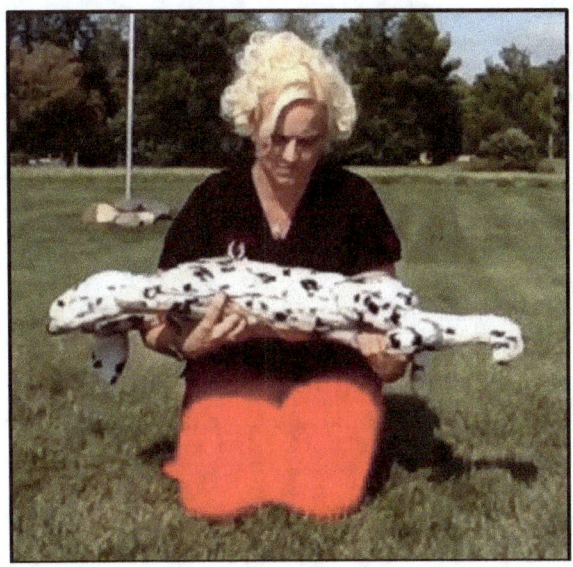

Using a Stretcher

Any solid flat surface can be used as a stretcher to transport a dog. A flat board must be used if a broken back or severe traumatic injury is suspected. In many cases, you can use a blanket or flat board as a stretcher. If you are using a blanket place one hand under the animal's chest and the other under its rear; carefully lift or slide the animal onto the blanket. Transport the animal to the veterinarian.

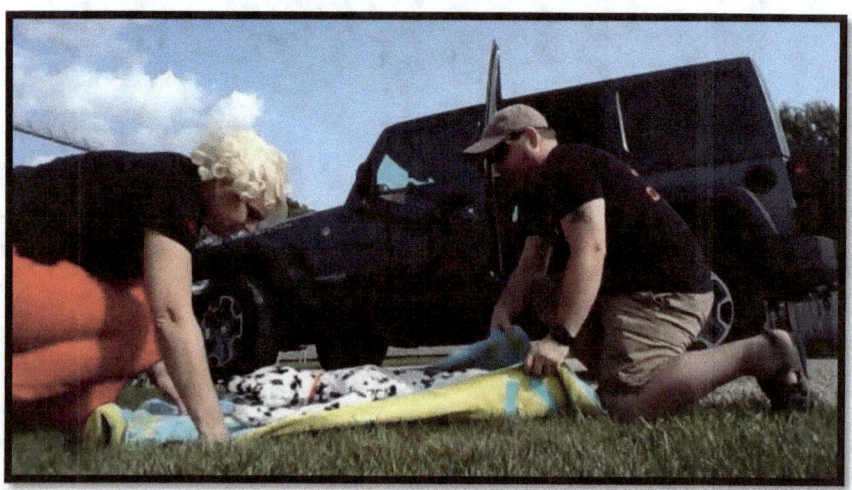

If you are using a flat board, depending on the size of the animal, use a table leaf, an ironing board, a large cutting board, or a removable bookshelf. Make sure whatever you use will fit in your car. Place 2 or 3 long strips of cloth or rope equidistant under the board, avoiding the area where the animal's neck will rest.

For a dog, place one hand under its chest and the other under its rear; carefully lift or slide the dog onto the board. Whenever possible it is good to tie the dog to the board to keep them from sliding off. As always, transport the dog to the veterinarian if they have sustained a serious injury.

If a cat needs a stretcher, use a blanket, a flat board, or a strong piece of cardboard. If you are using a blanket, place one hand under the cat's chest and the other hand under its rear. Carefully lift or slide the cat onto the blanket. Grasp each end of the blanket and lift. Try to keep the blanket taut to form a stretcher. You can also use a flat board or a strong piece of cardboard. Place two or three long strips of cloth or rope under the board, avoiding the area where the cat's neck will rest. Place one hand under the cat's chest and the other under its rear; carefully lift or slide the cat onto the board. Tie the cat to the board to prevent him or her from falling.

Safe Restraint and Handling of Dogs and Cats

Restraint positions for dogs and cats are utilized to keep the animal positioned to better evaluate them or move them from one place to another. We also use proper restraint to keep the people working with animals safe. Use caution when restraining any animal. Animals can be aggressive and reactive when in pain. You need to be aware of the animals' injuries before manipulating their body as this could injure them further and make their condition worse.

Dog Restraint

Make sure to observe the dog's body language as you approach them. Sometimes you can easily scoop a dog into your arms; when they are in pain that might not be the case, however. There are some common mistakes that you should try to avoid. Never put your face in the dog's face as you can easily get bitten. Do not expect an injured dog to behave the way it normally does; pain and fear can illicit many different behaviors that can cause harm to the caregiver. Depending on the situation and suspected injury, dogs can lay on their side as in the picture below on the right, or standing, such as the picture on the left.

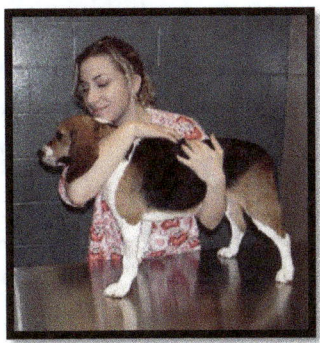 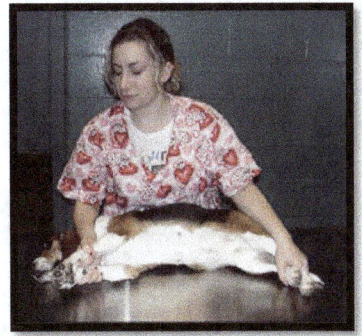

Applying a Gauze Muzzle to a Dog

An injured dog, no matter how gentle, has the propensity to bite when hurt or injured. Animals will not understand your intentions and may act out in a very dangerous manner. Any dog might think that what you are doing is what's causing it pain. Instinctively they may bite to protect themselves from further harm. An emergency muzzle can be a very useful tool and, if done correctly, can protect you from a dangerous bite. It can be made with a shoelace, string, leash, necktie, ace bandage, belt, or anything that is long enough to wrap around the dog's muzzle.

** DO NOT APPLY A MUZZLE TO A DOG THAT IS UNCONSCIOUS, VOMITING, HAVING DIFFICULTY BREATHING OR SEIZURING.

The following steps will instruct you how to place an emergency muzzle on a dog using a piece of rolled gauze:

Step 1. Use rolled gauze and cut a length long enough to wrap around the muzzle and tie behind the ears. Bring the center of the gauze up under the muzzle, then wrap the gauze around the top of the muzzle and bring back underneath.

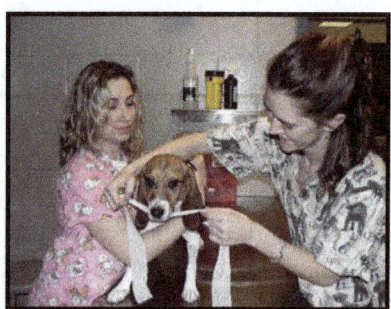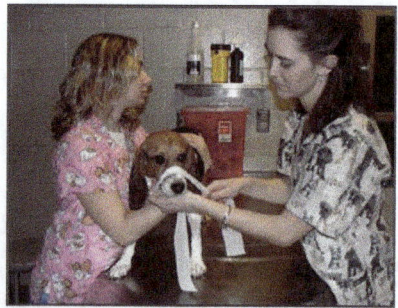

Step 2. Cross the gauze under the jaw and bring back behind the ears. Tie snuggly in a bow. Do not tie gauze in a knot because if the animal goes into distress then you will need to be able to remove it quickly.

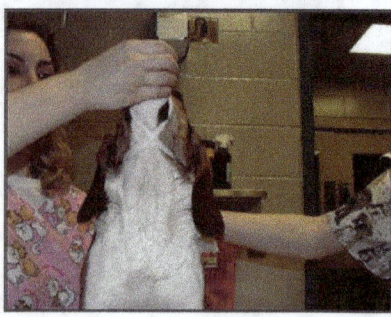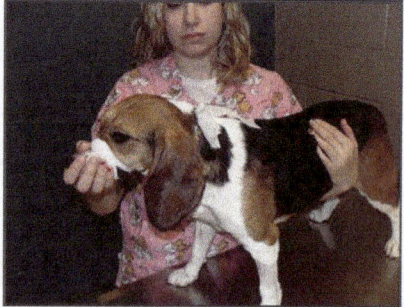

How to Use the Leash to Place an Emergency Muzzle

Sometimes when a dog gets hurt the injury is very painful. This may cause the dog to snap or bite you if you attempt to assist them. A safe way to protect yourself from harm while treating your dog is to place an emergency muzzle on them using a leash.

The following steps will instruct you how to put an emergency muzzle on with a leash.

1. Wrap the leash completely around the dog's muzzle right below its eyes.

2. Crisscross the leash under the neck and bring up behind the ears.

3. Slip the hand loop end through the base of the metal clip (not through the clip itself)

4. Pull the leash snug and adjust around the dog's head to make sure that the leash is keeping the mouth shut to prevent a bite. You can even clip the metal clasp on the leash to the dog's collar for extra stability.

5. Hold the leash tight and never leave a dog unattended with a muzzle on!

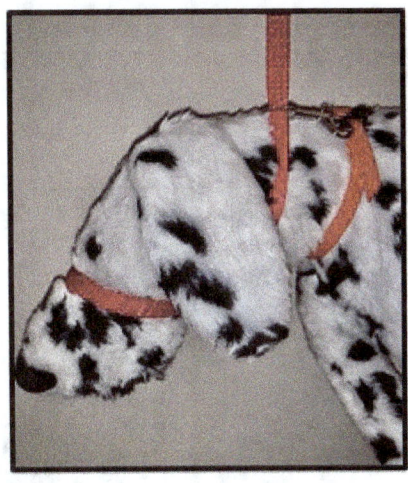

Cat Restraint

Cats tend to be more reactive than dogs, therefore it is especially important to never let your guard down. Cats also have scratching as a means of defense. With cats, less restraint is oftentimes better. Scruffing a cat (such as the picture below) is a quick and painless technique that you can use as long as you do not scruff the cat for very long. Scruffing is when you grip the loose skin behind the cat's neck in one hand.

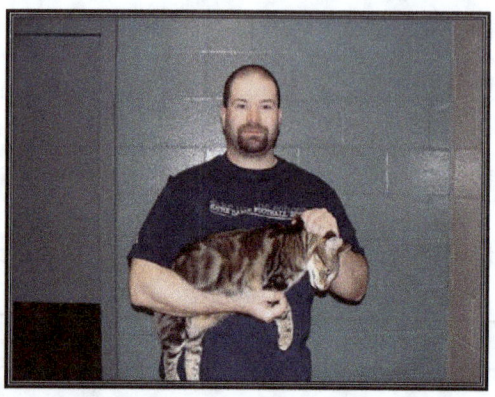

Towel Restraint for Cats

Towel restraint is useful when you must hold a cat still or move a cat that is actively trying to scratch you. Place a bath sized towel or pillowcase on a table or countertop. Put the cat in the center of the towel with the length of its body parallel to the shorter end of the towel. Pull one end up over the cat until it reaches the other side of the body. Apply firm pressure to the towel to keep it snug while folding the other side of the towel up and around the cat. The cat should look like a "kitty burrito".

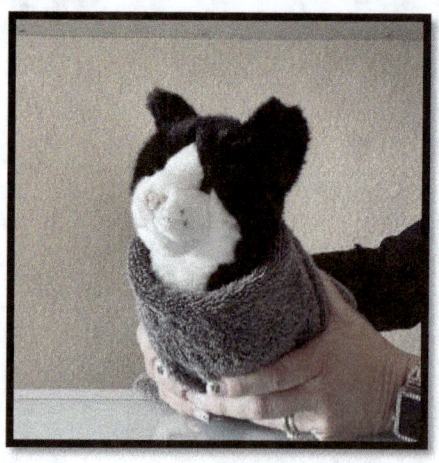

Triage

Triage is the art of assigning priority to emergency patients and their problems based on rapid assessment of historical and physical parameters. The triage should take about 5 minutes. The goal is to quickly identify patients with life-threatening problems so they can be treated immediately. If a patient requires immediate evaluation by a veterinarian, verbal permission or signed medical consent should be obtained from the owners that authorizes the appropriate emergency treatment (CPR, IV catheter, medication, radiographs, blood work, etc.) as quickly as possible. Perform a rapid, whole body exam looking for wounds, bruises (petechiae, purpura or ecchymosis), abdominal pain/distention and any other signs of debilitation. Wounds to the thorax or abdomen can be critical even if the patient appears stable on triage. [9]

How to be a Prepared in an Emergency

When handling a medical emergency for a pet you will likely need to bring an animal to the closest veterinary hospital. Prior to leaving for the vet you should do the following:

Call ahead, if possible- If at all call the vet when you are on your way. This can be extremely helpful as the veterinary staff can prepare for the pet's arrival by setting up equipment and medications that will be needed.

Try to collect all relevant information- Having the pet's breed, age, vaccination status, and any medications they are taking can be very important. Ideally the person bringing the pet should be able to answer questions about the pet's care and lifestyle.

Obvious Emergency
Life-threatening conditions
- Cardiopulmonary arrest
- Cyanosis/Severe respiratory distress
- Collapse/Unresponsive
- GDV (Gastric Dilatation Volvulus)/Dog with unproductive vomiting or abdominal distention
- Profuse blood loss
- Penetrating wound
- Severe trauma
- Heatstroke
- Shock

Strong Potential for Emergency

Conditions that will likely become life-threatening without treatment

- Difficulty breathing/Wheezing
- Allergic reactions
- Smoke inhalation
- Trouble walking or moving, neurologic problems
- Paralysis of hind limbs or all limbs
- Trauma: Large laceration; Hit by car; Puncture wound to head, neck, chest, or abdomen
- Electrocution
- Snakebite
- Eye injury
- A diabetic
- A puppy that is lethargic or not eating
- Dystocia/active labor
- Ingestion of toxic substance or foreign body
- Severe pain

Non-Emergent Triage

These situations are usually stable and present with minor complaints however animals are experiencing some type of pain and/or distress. There is still a problem that needs to be fixed. It is important to use low-stress handling techniques for animals. Safely obtain whatever vitals you are able and advise the veterinarian of the situation. Vitals can be obtained at the same time as the vet's exam to reduce stress.

When to Get to the Vet in an Emergency

Triage Level	Amount of Time that You Have to Get an Animal to a Vet clinic	Examples of medical emergencies at this level
1	Immediately	Cardiac Arrest, GDV, Heatstroke
2	<10 minutes	Severe Trauma, Allergic reactions causing swelling in the face
3	<1 hour	Dehydration, trouble moving
4	1-2 hours	Vomiting, wounds
5	1-4 hours	Coughing, minor wound

Table Reference: Triage and assessment of the emergency patient - WSAVA 2017 Congress - Vin. Powered By VIN. (n.d.). Retrieved January 15, 2023, from https://www.vin.com/apputil/content

Physical Examination

The physical exam is a series of observations that are made to determine the severity of a victim's medical condition and what approach for first aid should be made. It is important to be thorough but as quick as possible. This animal does not have much time so finding out what first aid it needs is imperative. Before starting a hands-on exam, stand back and look at the pet. Look at the animal's posture, breathing, activity level, and general appearance. Four different observations are used to conduct a physical exam. These include visual inspection, palpation (sense of touch), percussion(tapping on areas of the body), and auscultation(listening to) The use of these senses helps us determine any abnormalities. Clinical examination can be undergone by taking vital sign, general clinical examination, and systemic examination of animals.

The following are the parts of a general physical exam:

- Listening to an animal's lungs and heart

- Checking the cat or dog's stance, gait, and weight

- Examining the pet's eyes for signs of excessive tearing, discharge, redness, cloudiness, or eyelid issues

- Checking the pet's coat for overall condition, abnormal hair loss, or dandruff

- Examining the pet's nails and feet for damage or signs of a more serious health condition

- Looking at the pet's ears for signs of bacterial infection, ear mites, or wax

- Examining the condition of the pet's teeth for any indications of periodontal disease, damage, or decay

- Checking a pet's skin for a handful of problems such as parasites, dryness, lumps, and bumps (specifically in skin folds)

- Feeling the pet's abdomen to access the internal organs to see if they appear normal and to check for signs of discomfort

- Feeling along a cat or dog's body (palpating) for hints of illness including swelling, evidence of lameness (such as limited range of motion), and signs of pain

It's important for every pet owner and animal professional to know the basics when it comes to an animal's vital signs. Vital signs are measurements of the body's most basic functions. Obtaining vital signs can help assess the pet's physical condition in an emergency situation and better prepare for sharing important information with a veterinarian. The three main vitals to assess are: heart rate/pulse, respiratory rate, and temperature.

BODY TEMPERATURE: Normal = Dog- 100.2-102.5 and Cats- 100.5- 102.5 degrees Fahrenheit

The internal body temperature for dogs and cats is taken rectally. It is best to use a digital thermometer that is safe for pets. Thermometers that are safe for pets have a flexible tip so that the thermometer does not injure the pet when it is placed in the rectum and take no more than 20 seconds to get a reading.

To take a pet's temperature, first coat the thermometer with a lubricant such as petroleum gel or baby oil. Next, gently insert the thermometer about one inch into the dog or cat's anus and wait for results.

HEART RATE:
Dog: Normal = 70-120 beats/minute dependent on size - normal values for canine heart rates depend on their size. A heart rate of 140 may be normal in a Yorkshire terrier but would be abnormal for a Mastiff.

Cat: Normal = 120-140 beats/minute. Trends should be monitored over a period when nursing critical patients. A change in a patient's heart rate may indicate an issue.

CIRCULATION: Check for a heartbeat and note the heart rate and rhythm. Palpate the femoral or another distal arterial pulse. Feel the gums, ears, and extremities to see if they are cool. See if there is any evidence of bleeding.

PULSES: Normal pulses are strong and regular. The pulse is the difference between systolic and diastolic pressures. A strong pulse may not mean the animal has adequate blood pressure. Pulses are located on the inside of the thigh (femoral), the top of the foot (pedal), or the underside of the tail. The pulse strength helps you to evaluate perfusion. The pulse will deteriorate with worsening shock, dehydration, or heart function. Normal pulses are steady and even, beating in a constant pattern with the same strength to each beat, and will disappear under moderate pressure.

An irregular pulse may be due to sinus arrhythmia or heart disease. Weak pulses are slightly stronger than thready pulses and will disappear with light pressure. A weak pulse signifies a decreased difference between systolic and diastolic pressure that may be due to low cardiac output. Thready pulses are not easily felt, and may feel like a small fine thread under the finger and will disappear with slight pressure. A bounding pulse feels full and spring-like on palpation and will not disappear under moderate pressure. A bounding pulse may be due to low peripheral resistance, increased cardiac output, and increased stroke volume.

How to obtain a heart rate on an animal

*Place your stethoscope on the left side of the animal, just behind the point of the elbow, to listen to the heart beating.

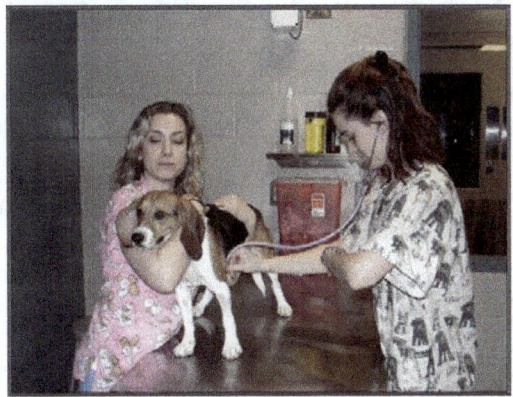

*Place two fingers on the inner thigh where the leg meets the body to feel the femoral pulse. Put your index finger right below the ankle on either the top or bottom of the paw (this is the most difficult location to find a heart rate)

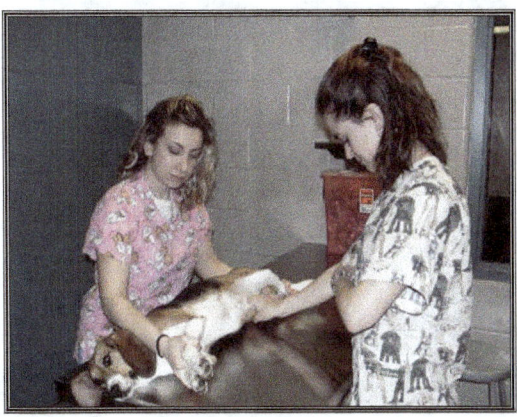

*Once you find a location count the beats in 15 seconds and then multiply by 4 and this will give you the BPM or beats per minute.

RESPIRATION: Dog: Normal = 18-34 breaths/minute and Cat: Normal = 16-40 breaths/minute, with no visible effort. The respiratory rate and effort are signs of how well the animal is breathing and can be indicators of problems. Monitor the animal for changes in its respiratory rate or effort. These changes can be life-threatening.

MUCOUS MEMBRANE COLOR: Normal = pink Abnormal color includes bright red, white, blue, or yellow. All four of these gum colors indicate that there is a serious problem. **CAPILLARY REFILL TIME (CRT):** Normal = 1-2 seconds. Mucous m membrane color and capillary refill time (CRT) serve to evaluate perfusion, oxygenation, and some underlying diseases. Mucous membrane color is assessed by lifting the upper lip and quickly pressing on the gums with finger to push the blood out of the tissue, then removing your finger and counting the number of seconds it takes for the color to return. This should normally take 1 to 2 seconds.

In a life-threatening emergency, you may also look deeper at the following:

AIRWAY: Check for a patent airway. Ensure the mouth and throat are clear of obstructions.

BREATHING: Observe if the animal is breathing and if they are breathing effectively. Note if there is any extra effort taken. Determine if there is a need for supplemental oxygen. Listen to the lungs' sounds. Listen to different areas to see if the sounds are different. Check the color of the mucous membranes and the capillary refill time. Note any abnormal signs/sounds. Respiratory distress may present with no chest wall movement, nasal flaring, open mouth breathing, head and neck extension, exaggerated effort, and paradoxical breathing.

Emergencies Requiring Immediate Attention

Most emergencies require some type of veterinary attention. The purpose of first aid is to be able to administer emergency care to a pet that is experiencing a severe injury or condition which may become life-threatening. First Aid can also include more minor injuries by which the first aid will minimize the severity of the condition until veterinary intervention is obtained. An emergency can be anything from a small wound to something as urgent as an animal that is unconscious. Throughout this next section, you will see a list of medical emergencies that will need the attention of a veterinary hospital immediately.

Zoonoses are infections and/or diseases that are passed from animals to people. Such conditions can present a public health concern. Zoonoses can be caused by a range of disease pathogens such as viruses, bacteria, fungi, and parasites. Of 1,415 pathogens known to infect humans, 61% were zoonotic and transmissible from an animal. These diseases can be contracted via urine, feces, respiratory secretions, scratches, and bites from the animal or insects.

Most of the zoonotic or infectious diseases listed below are rare, but pet owners do need to be aware of them:

Anthrax
Cat scratch fever
Eastern Equine
Encephalomyelitis
Ercherichia coli
Giardiasis
Leptospirosis
Listeriosis
Lyme Disease

Plague
Psittacosis
Rabies
Ringworm
Salmonellosis
Tetanus
Tick Paralysis
Toxoplsmosis
Tuberculosis

Some ways that you can protect yourself from contracting a zoonotic disease is to place a barrier between you and the animal, do not handle food and do not touch your eyes, nose or mouth until you can wash your hands after touching an animal. If sharp objects are involved, use extreme caution as cutting yourself with a contaminated object can potential transmit a zoonotic disease. In any case of exposure to a zoonotic disease seek medical treatment immediately.

Allergic Reactions

Signs of an allergic reaction can include anything from itchiness, hives, swelling on face, redness and even collapse and shock. Like people, many pets have allergies to common things pollen, food and residues, etc. Allergies are especially common in dogs, however, there are some allergic reactions that can cause the airway to swell shut therefore becoming a life-threatening emergency.

Allergies are immune responses to substances like pollen, dust, food, or fur that can cause discomfort and illness. Over time, exposure to those substances, called allergens, can sensitize the immune system, and cause a harmful over-reaction. Itchiness is the most common symptom of allergic reactions. If left untreated this itchiness can cause sores, hot spots and skin infections. Animals having an allergic reaction to something requires some basic first aid. First try to identify the allergen and remove the animal from the allergen. Next, wipe any residue, pollen, etc. off the animal. You can use a mild shampoo, such as an oatmeal shampoo, to wash the animal if necessary. You can also put a cool compress on any itchy areas of the skin. Always consult a veterinarian before giving any antihistamines to the animal.

While more uncommon, severe allergies can cause a condition called anaphylaxis. Anaphylaxis can be caused by insect stings, medications, vaccines, and certain foods. Anaphylaxis shows such symptoms as diarrhea, vomiting, shock, seizures, com, and then death. This type of allergic reaction is a life-threatening emergency. It needs veterinary attention immediately. A veterinary clinic has the necessary medications and equipment to help an animal in anaphylaxis. Keep animals calm and monitor their breathing and pulse while en route to the clinic. If the animal stops breathing be prepared to begin CPR. The image below show hives on the skin of a dog.

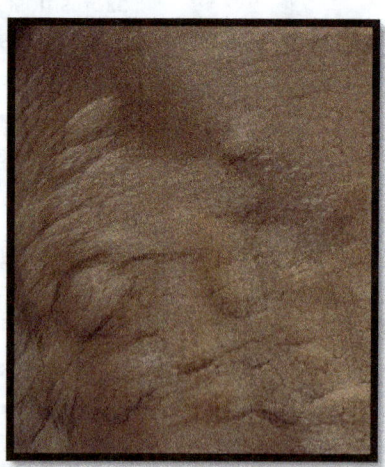

Anxiety with Fireworks and Loud Noises

Pets are more sensitive than we are to loud noises, flashing lights, and strong smells. This can be caused by events like thunderstorms and fireworks.

On the Fourth of July, and other days people are likely to set off fireworks, or during thunderstorms, it's best to leave pets safely indoors, preferably with a radio or TV turned on or a fan to soften jarring noises. Even pets who usually spend a lot of time outdoors should be brought inside. Pets will feel more secure if they have a certain area that they know is safe for them and they can relax in. For some dogs this might be their crate, for others it might be a corner that they go to often to escape the hustle and bustle of everyday life.

Make sure pets have some sort of identification in case they escape from the yard. Microchipping is the safest and most reliable way to identify a pet. Collars with ID tags also help in case they do get out and become lost. This can save a lot of time in getting them back to their owners quickly if someone finds them.

Times of the year when fireworks are common is also a time for parties and BBQs. Be careful of what pets eat. They can get foreign objects lodged in their stomach/intestines such as corn cobs, chicken bones, rawhides, rope toys, pieces of bones, and string and hair elastics in cats too.

Protect pets from heat stroke. If dogs are running around in the yard having fun, make sure it is not too hot out. If it's hot, try to avoid midday play from 10a-3p when it is the hottest, or simply wait until the sun goes down. Take breaks often, even if it is not hot, by putting them inside and giving them plenty of access to water. Breeds such as Bulldogs, Pugs, Puggles, Pekingese, French Bulldogs, Boston Terriers, or any other brachycephalic "squished-faced" dog, should primarily be in areas that are cool.

There are a variety of medications, supplements and calming vests that can help reduce dog's stress and anxiety from fireworks, and a veterinarian (or a board-certified veterinary behaviorist) is the best person to help determine which one, or ones, are best for pets. Every pet, and every situation, is different therefore a licensed veterinary professional is the best to consult.

Bloat (Gastric Dilatation Volvulus)

Bloat is an extremely serious condition that should be considered a life-threatening emergency. Dog owners and animal professionals that work with dogs must contact their veterinarians immediately if they suspect that a dog has bloat. Dogs can die of bloat within several hours. Even with treatment, as many as 25-33% of dogs with GDV die.

The gastric dilatation is one part of the condition and the volvulus or torsion is the second part. In bloat (dilatation), due to several different and sometimes unknown reasons, the stomach fills up with air and puts pressure on the other organs and diaphragm. The pressure on the diaphragm makes it difficult for the dog to breathe.

The air-filled stomach also compresses large veins in the abdomen, thus preventing blood from returning to the heart. Filled with air, the stomach can easily rotate on itself, thus pinching off its blood supply. Once this rotation (volvulus) occurs and the blood supply is cut off, the stomach begins to die, and the entire blood supply is disrupted, and the animal's condition begins to deteriorate very rapidly.

Not all dogs that have a gas buildup and resultant dilatation develop the more serious and life-threatening volvulus. However, almost all dogs that have a volvulus develop it because of a dilatation. There are several breeds that have a higher occurrence of bloat than others. Large breed dogs with deep, narrow chests are more likely to develop bloat.

Some of those breeds include:

- Great Dane
- Saint Bernard
- Weimaraner
- Irish Setter
- Gordon Setter
- Standard Poodle

The most obvious signs of bloat are abdominal distention (swollen belly) and vomiting where the animal does not throw anything up. Other signs include restlessness, abdominal pain, and rapid shallow breathing. Profuse salivation may indicate severe pain.

If the dog's condition continues to deteriorate, especially if volvulus has occurred, the dog may go into shock and become pale, have a weak pulse, a rapid heart rate, and eventually collapse. A dog with gastric dilatation without volvulus can show all these signs, but the more severe signs are likely to occur in dogs with both dilatation and volvulus.

Veterinarians suspect that certain factors such as drinking too much water, gulping down food quickly, and exercising too soon before or after eating can lead to bloat. If you suspect that your dog has bloat you need to get them to a veterinarian as quickly as possible. There is nothing you can do at home and getting them prompt emergency veterinary care will be the only way to hopefully save their life. Try to keep the animal as still as possible.

If you suspect that your dog may be at risk of bloat there may be some options to help prevent an episode. Below is a list of suggestions:

- Feeding several small meals each day
- Do not feed dogs from an elevated food bowl
- Avoiding dry kibble
- Offering water at all times
- Trying to reduce stress, especially around feeding time

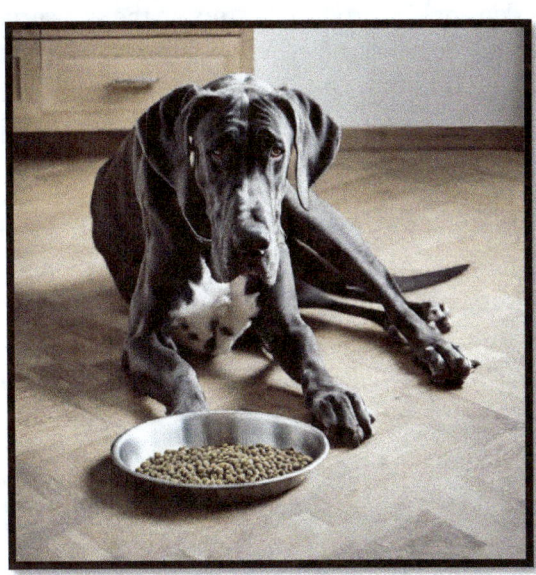

Dogs especially large breeds such as Great Danes
should always be fed from a bowl on the floor to prevent bloat

Burns

Burns are often profoundly serious and can be caused by a variety of sources. Some of these sources can include electrical equipment, hot water or liquids and chemicals. It is important that immediate first aid be provided to a burn to lessen its severity. Burns will require immediate medical attention from a licensed veterinarian as they can cause deep tissue damage, infection and in extreme cases shock.

Symptoms of Burns- Animals with first-degree burns generally will show signs of pain such as vocalization. With most first degree burns the skin will remain intact. Second-degree and third-degree burns, on the other hand, are far more serious. The skin is either partly or completely burned. In these situations, check for signs of shock and provide immediate first aid as outlined in the chart on the next page below.

Categories of Burns

1st degree: Superficial partial thickness wounds - These burns involve only the top layer of skin. The symptoms are generally limited to minor pain and redness. An example of a superficial partial-thickness burn is mild sunburn. 1st-degree burns heal quickly and generally do not require extra care.

2nd degree: Deep partial thickness wounds - These burns involve the deeper layers of skin and will produce blisters on the skin surface. They are more painful, introduce a risk of infection and take longer to heal. 2nd-degree burns require veterinary attention.

3rd degree: Full-thickness wounds - These burns involve complete destruction of all skin layers. Charring is seen. There is usually no sensation left in the area. With the loss of the skin's protective layer, the animal is now highly susceptible to bacterial infection. Circulation to the burned area is compromised, as is the immune response. In addition, burns of this type greatly affect the pet's electrolyte balance. These burns are the most dangerous and life-threatening; they require immediate and extensive veterinary care.

Types of Burns

Chemical burns- Burns caused by chemical agents may also be difficult to recognize because the pet's hair coat may hide the burn. Chemical burns are generally erosive and necrotic (leading to the death of tissue) in nature. These burns are usually 2nd degree but maybe 3rd degree. Again, it may take up to 48 hours for the full extent of the burn to be apparent.

To avoid being bitten while administering first aid you may have to muzzle your pet. Make sure the area you are working in is well ventilated and if the burn is from a dry chemical, brush away as much of the substance as possible. Be sure to protect the mouth, nose, and eyes of both yourself and the pet while washing the contaminated area with large amounts of warm (not Hot!) flowing water. Protect yourself with appropriate safety equipment.

If the chemical is in the pet's eyes, flush with clean water or sterile saline for 15-20 minutes. Do not apply any ointments or butter-like substances. Do not apply ice to the burn and carefully transport the animal to your veterinarian! If possible, bring the chemical container with you.

Electrical burns- Electrical burns are mostly found in the mouth as a result of the animal chewing on an electric cord. The lips, gums, tongue, and palate (roof of the mouth) may be involved. Electrical burns are also erosive and necrotic in nature. There is usually one central area of necrosis (dead tissue) surrounded by areas of varying tissue damage. Dogs are more often affected.

If the animal is unconscious due to an electrocution, CPR should be started immediately if the animal is in cardiac arrest. If the animal is still conscious, you can carefully rinse the burned area with cool water. Transport the pet to a veterinarian as quickly as possible and watch for signs of shock.

Thermal Burns- This type of burn results from flames or hot surfaces and are usually obvious from their onset, however they can take 24-48 hours to fully appear. Thermal burns are usually 2nd or 3rd degree burns. They are very painful and can cause significant tissue damage.

Electric heating pads should NEVER be used on pets! Burns caused by commonly used items such as heating pads or hot-air cage dryers may be difficult to diagnosis. The tissue damage is typically hidden by the animal's fur. It may take 24-48 hours for the full extent of the burn to appear. The burned area will appear hard and dry.

Burns of this nature result in a 1st or 2nd degree burn. First extinguish all flames, or if electricity is involved, make sure the power is turned off. To avoid being bitten you may have to muzzle the animal. Apply a cool water compress with a clean (sterile) cloth. This may prevent the burn from penetrating deeper into the tissues. Change the compress frequently and keep the site cool and wet.

Do not break any blisters that may have formed and do not apply any ointments or butter-like substances to the burn. Do not apply ice to the burn and carefully transport the animal to your veterinarian!

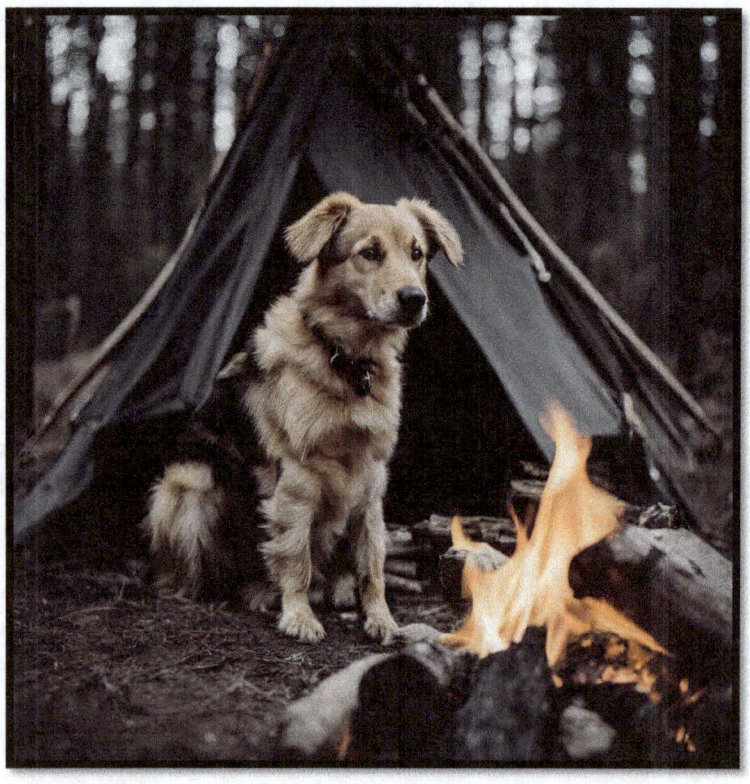

Great care should always be taken when pets are around fire,
hot pavement and other surfaces that could cause severe burns

Choking

If an animal is suffocating, it will often panic. A dog may paw at its mouth if something is lodged, though this does not necessarily mean it is choking. Another suspicious sign of choking is an unresponsive or unconscious dog; in these cases, check the throat and mouth for foreign objects. Carefully open the animal's mouth and if you see any objects in the oral cavity use your pinky finger and do a side-to-side sweep to try and dislodge the object. If you can see the object but are unable to put your fingers in the animal's mouth you can try to remove it with a pair of salad tongs, tweezers, needle nose pliers, etc.

If the object is not visible, you may need to perform back blows or abdominal thrusts to dislodge the object from the animal's airway. Use the following steps for an animal that is small enough that you can hold them on your forearm such as the picture below. Hold the animal on your arm with its head facing down, allowing gravity to help draw the object out. Next, use the palm of your hand and hit the animal between the shoulder blades 4 times. After the 4th time, recheck the animal's airway to see if the object has come up far enough to reach it and if it has not, repeat the preceding steps again.

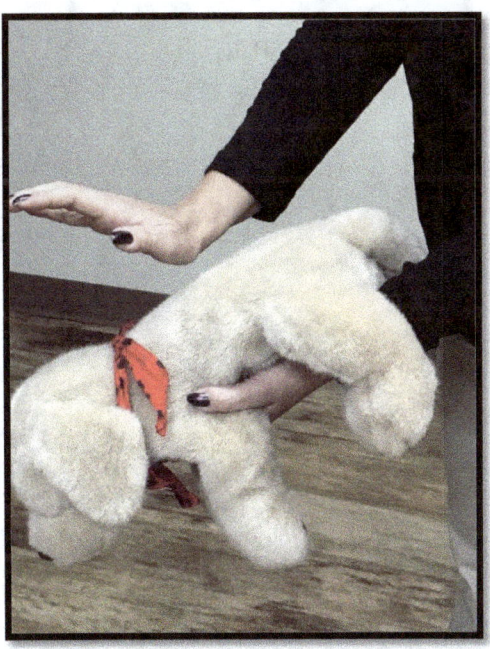

The image above demonstrates how you would hold an animal to perform back blows

For an animal that is too large to support on your, arm you will need to perform abdominal thrusts to attempt to dislodge the object. Stand over the animal and put your arms around the animal's abdomen. Pull upward forcefully 4 times, then check the airway again. If the object has become dislodged make sure to remove it from the oral cavity. If the object is still obstructed, repeat 4 more thrusts. Repeat until the object has been dislodged. Once you have removed the object, check for breathing. If the animal is not breathing begin CPR.

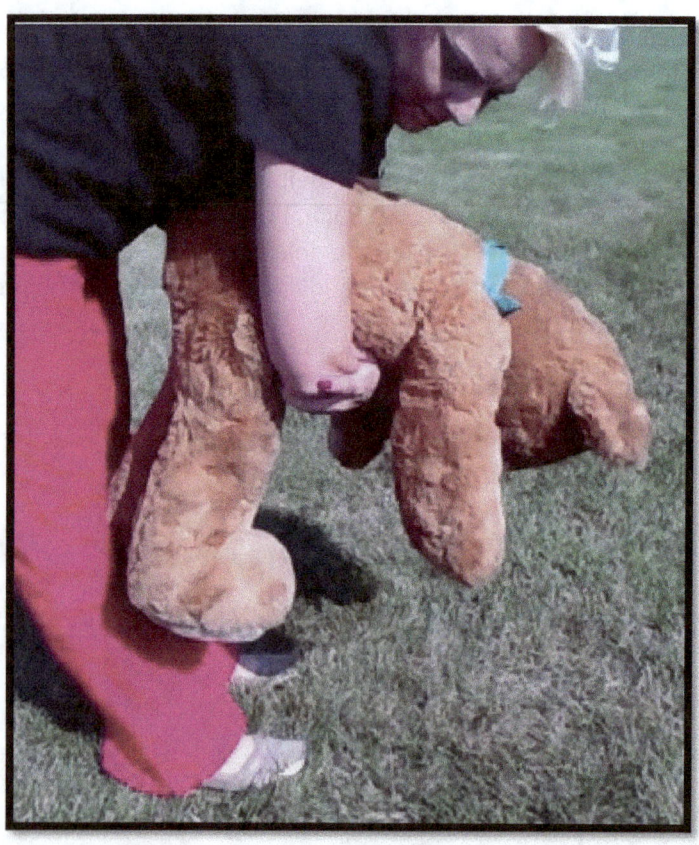

When performing abdominal thrusts wrap your arms around the dog's abdomen and pull upwards

Difficulty Breathing

As an animal inhales, fresh air moves through the nose (or mouth), pharynx, and larynx to the trachea. The trachea carries the air to the bronchi, which in turn supply the lungs. Air exchange occurs in the alveoli and the used air follows the opposite path of new air: passing into the bronchi, into the trachea, through the larynx and pharynx, and finally exiting through the nose or mouth. Breathing is relatively simple and is accomplished by the actions of the rib muscles (intercostals) and the movement of a great internal muscle called the diaphragm.

The diaphragm muscle separates the chest, containing the heart and lungs, from the abdomen, which holds the intestines, stomach, liver, bladder, etc. As this powerful muscle moves toward the abdomen, it creates a negative pressure and pulls fresh air and oxygen into the lungs, causing the dog to breathe in (inhale). The chest cavity surrounding the lungs is a vacuum, thus allowing the lungs to inflate easily when the dog inhales. When the muscle moves forward (towards the animal's head), it causes the lungs to compress and force air out (exhale), thus ridding the body of used air. *Foster DVM, Race. "Respiratory System: Anatomy & Function in Dogs." Pet Education. N.p., n.d. Web. 23 Jan. 2017.*

There are many reasons an animal may have difficulty breathing such as shock, allergic reactions, collapsed lungs, pneumonia, and choking. When an animal's breathing is labored, it takes much more effort for them to inhale and exhale. The animal's breathing patterns may change, and you might notice symptoms such as gasping, wheezing, or struggling to draw in air.

Cats that are open-mouth breathing, or animals with blue mucous membranes, need to be rushed to a veterinary clinic immediately. You should never muzzle an animal that is having difficulty breathing as it could cause them to go into respiratory arrest and stop breathing.

Respiratory arrest is the cessation of breathing due to the failure of the lungs to function effectively. Apnea is the cessation of breathing. Prolonged apnea refers to an animal who has stopped breathing for a long period of time. If the heart muscle contraction is intact, the condition is known as respiratory arrest. An abrupt stop of pulmonary gas exchange lasting for more than five minutes may damage vital organs, especially the brain, possibly permanently. Lack of oxygen to the brain causes loss of consciousness. Brain injury is likely if respiratory arrest goes untreated for more than three minutes, and death is almost certain if left untreated for more than five minutes.

The gums in the animal's mouth should be pink as you see in the top picture below. The shade of pink can vary, but in general, you are looking for a pink color. This means that there is normal blood flow to the tissues with adequate oxygenation. When the gum color becomes pale (as in the bottom picture), white or blue it usually means there is not enough blood and/or oxygen getting to the body. Bright red gums might indicate toxicity or hyperthermia and yellow gums can indicate organ failure.

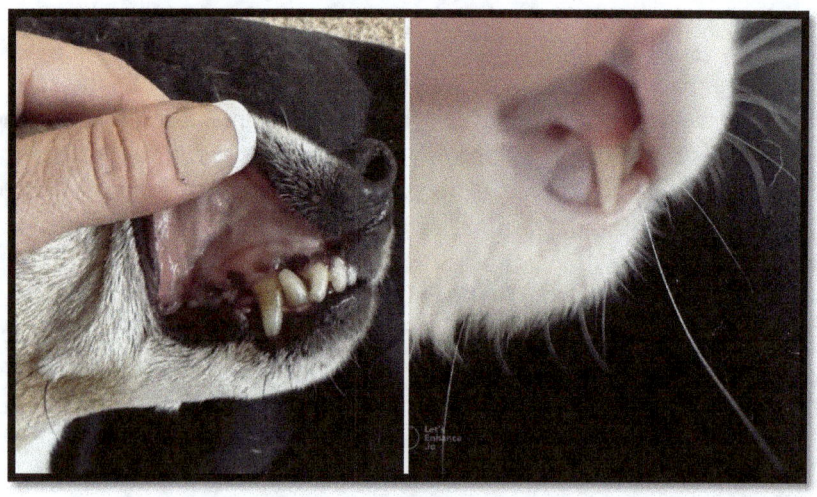

Gums in the mouth of a dog (left) or cat (right) should appear pink as pictured above.

Drowning

Dogs, more than cats, generally love water. Most dogs have a natural ability to swim and enjoy time in the water. Even though by nature they are good swimmers, situations of drowning can still happen. Inhalation of fluid can be caused by owner negligence, young dogs that are not experienced swimmers, weak, elderly animals, or trauma. Near-drowning is when an event occurs that involves prolonged submersion or inhalation of fluid such as water or vomit. Once the fluid fills the lungs the animal is no longer able to breathe and carbon dioxide begins to build in the bloodstream.

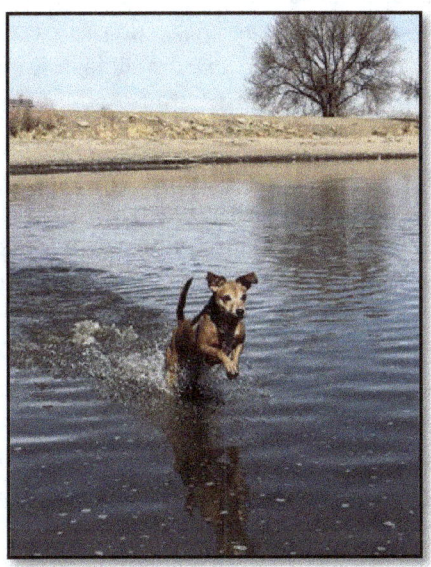

These are the phases in a typical drowning:

- Breath-holding and swimming motion
- Water aspiration
- Choking
- Struggling for air
- Cessation of movement
- Unconsciousness then Death

When you come across an animal drowning, safely remove the animal from the water first and then check for consciousness. If the animal is not breathing, lift the animal by the hind legs to allow water to come out of the nose or mouth. Lay the animal down on either side with the head lowered. Go through the series of A,B,C before performing CPR or rescue breathing. Get to a veterinary clinic as soon as possible.

Hyperthermia

Hyperthermia is an elevation in body temperature that is above the generally accepted normal range. Although normal values for dogs and cats vary slightly, it usually is accepted that a body temperature above 103° F (39° C) is abnormal. Heat stroke, meanwhile, is a form of non-fever hyperthermia that occurs when heat-dissipating mechanisms of the body cannot accommodate excessive external heat. Typically associated with the temperature of 106° F (41°C) or higher without signs of inflammation, heat stroke can lead to multiple organ dysfunction. On hot days, the animal can become overheated and lethargic very quickly, especially if they are participating in a lot of outdoor activity, such as running. The animal's tongue may hang out and it will pant extremely fast. Remember, cats that are open-mouth breathing are in a much more severe state of distress.

Bring the animal indoors or in the shade and provide them with water. Keep them in a cool place and monitor them closely. You can also pour cool (*not cold*) water over the animal to help reduce its temperature. DO NOT submerge them in water, this can cause them to go into shock. You can also wrap ice packs in a towel and place them on the animal. If you are out hiking or somewhere where you might not be able to get inside quickly, you can place the animal's feet in a stream or other water source. One should never leave an animal in a car in the summer; however, if you see an animal in a hot car call your local authorities before taking matters into your own hands. There are laws concerning breaking and entering a vehicle even if there is an animal inside. The internal body temperature starting to rise within 15 minutes is a good sign. Continue to monitor the animal for signs of distress and then transport them to a veterinary hospital. Other signs that your animal might be experiencing heat stroke are fast heart rate, red gums, vomiting or diarrhea, and seizures.

Hypothermia is a medical condition that is characterized by an abnormally low body temperature and has three phases: mild, moderate, and severe. Mild hypothermia is classified as a body temperature of 90 - 99°F (or 32 - 35°C), moderate hypothermia at 82 - 90°F (28 - 32°C), and severe hypothermia is any temperature less than 82°F (28°C). Hypothermia occurs when an animal's body is no longer able to maintain normal temperature, causing a depression of the central nervous system (CNS). It may also affect heart and blood flow (cardiovascular), breathing (respiratory), and the immune system. An irregular heartbeat, trouble breathing, and impaired consciousness to the point of coma may result. Dogs do love to play in the snow so providing a nice warm coat and paw protection can be helpful as well.

Hypothermia

Hypothermia symptoms vary with the level of severity. Mild hypothermia is evident through weakness, shivering, and lack of mental alertness. Moderate hypothermia reveals characteristics such as muscle stiffness, low blood pressure, a stupor-like state and shallow, slow breathing. Characteristics of severe hypothermia are fixed and dilated pupils, inaudible heartbeat, difficulty breathing, and coma. Mild hypothermia may be treated passively, with thermal insulation and blankets to prevent further heat loss, while moderate hypothermia requires active external re-warming. This includes the use of external heat sources, such as radiant heat or heating pads, which can be applied to the animal's torso to warm its "core." A protective layer should be placed between the animal's skin and the heat source to avoid burns. For severe hypothermia, invasive core warming will be necessary, such as the administration of warm water enemas and warm intravenous (IV) fluids.

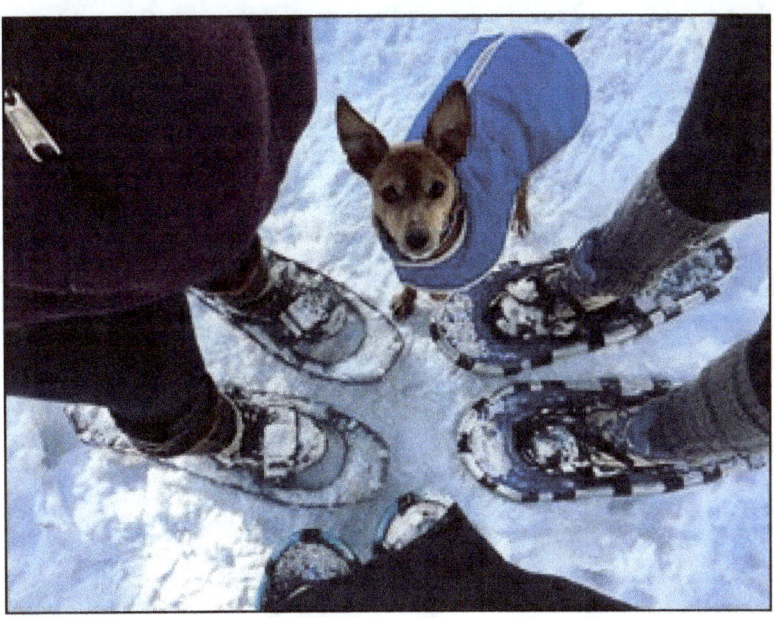

Dehydration

Dehydration is when there is a lack of water in the body. This can be serious and potentially life-threatening for pets. Water is a vital nutrient in the diet of dogs and cats and maintaining a proper daily fluid level is essential for life. 80% of your pet's body is made up of water. All biologic processes including circulation, digestion and waste removal utilizes water.

Dehydration occurs when fluid levels drop less than normal. This can happen either with reduced water intake or increased fluid loss. Fluid loss can happen in hot weather or with vomiting and diarrhea.

Symptoms of dehydration include dry mouth, depression, sunken eyes, and lethargy. If you suspect an animal is dehydrated, gently pull up on the skin between the animal's shoulder blades. This is called a "skin tent" test. In animals with normal hydration, the skin snaps back down against the animal's body quickly. If the skin stays up like a tent, then that is an indication of dehydration. Carefully offer water to the animal. Make sure the water is not too cold. It is best not to offer sports drinks or other electrolyte waters to the pet. These waters contain a large amount of sugar that is not good for pets. Be sure to seek veterinary care for any pet that is suspected of being dehydrated.

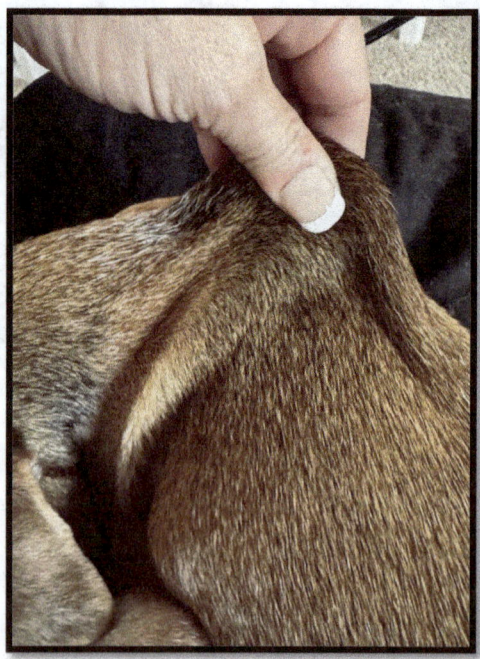

Skin Turgor test is when you pull up on an animal's skin and make a tent as seen in the picture above. If the skin stays up it means the animal might be dehydrated

You can always help to prevent dehydration by providing clean water and change it frequently to ensure freshness. Also, do not forget to wash a pet's water bowl every day to prevent bacteria from forming. Monitor the pet's water intake. Generally, dogs and cats need at least one ounce of water for each pound of body weight per day. If a pet is not drinking an adequate amount of water, seek veterinary advice. Monitoring water intake is especially important if a pet is recovering from diarrhea, vomiting or other illnesses.

Some other things that can be done are to purchase a water bowl with a weighted bottom to prevent a dog from knocking it over. Bring extra water when traveling or exercising with a dog. If you notice a pet is drinking less than usual, check its mouth for sores or other foreign objects, such as burrs or sticks. Avoid chaining a dog outside, since they may get tangled up, preventing them from accessing their water bowl. Keep the toilet lid closed to interrupt a dog's efforts to turn the bowl, which can be a source of bacteria, into a water fountain.

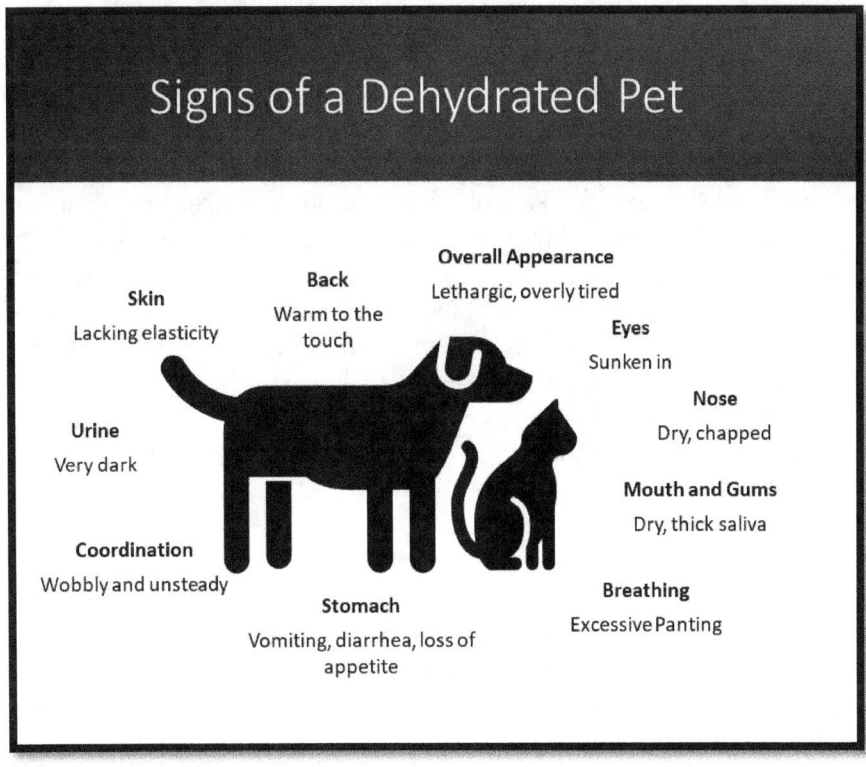

Poisons and Toxins

A poison is any substance with an inherent property that tends to destroy life or impair health. A toxin is any poison produced by an organism and including the bacterial toxins that are the causative agents of tetanus, diphtheria, etc., and such plant and animal toxins as ricin and snake venom. Symptoms of poisoning depend on which poison/toxin the animal encountered. They can include depression, weakness, trouble breathing, vomiting, facial and paw swelling, nausea, vomiting, diarrhea, abdominal pain, seizures, loss of coordination and disorientation, increased water intake and increased urination, excitation, salivation, foaming at the mouth, drooling, shallow respiration, collapsing, pale mucous membranes, coughing and swollen joints.

With most toxins, you can induce vomiting within 20 minutes of ingesting a poisonous item. It is important to speak to a veterinary professional for correct instructions on how to induce vomiting. Some toxins are absorbed so quickly or cause corrosive injury, that inducing vomiting is not recommended. If a dog is brachycephalic, or has a history of cardiovascular disease or seizures, it is not recommended to induce vomiting at home as this can lead to aspiration pneumonia and aggravate the dog's current health issues.

Unexpired 3% Hydrogen Peroxide can be used to induce vomiting in dogs. It should never be used in cats due to it causing hemorrhagic gastritis. Dogs can be given a dose of 1 teaspoon per 10 pounds, not to exceed 3 tablespoons. The best way to induce vomiting at home is to first feed the dog a few treats or small amount of their kibble. Hydrogen Peroxide can be administered using a syringe or turkey baster. Run the dog around afterwards, as this agitates the stomach and helps to induce vomiting. After 10 minutes, if vomiting has not occurred, a second dose of Hydrogen Peroxide can be given as long as the total given does not exceed 3 tablespoons.

Over the counter medications like Tylenol, Ibuprofen, and Aleve are not safe to give dogs and cats as pain relievers. They metabolize things different than humans. Tylenol will cause liver damage while Ibuprofen and Aleve cause bleeding stomach ulcers and kidney failure. Other common household foods such as grapes, raisins, garlic, onions, and chocolate also pose toxicity concerns. Grapes and raisins cause kidney failure while garlic and onions cause damage to red blood cells so they are not able to transport oxygen effectively.

The darker the chocolate the greater the toxicity risk. The toxic component in chocolate is Theobromine. High enough doses of Theobromine cause GI upset, cardiovascular changes, and central nervous symptom signs.

Many household plants pose toxicity risks and it is important to research which ones are safe before having the around your pets. For example, lilies are deadly to cats as they cause kidney failure. Just licking pollen or ingesting water that a lily has sat in is enough to cause kidney failure.

Rodenticides are commonly put out to control rodent populations, but these active ingredients will poison and kill dogs and cats the same as rodents. If they are put out, it is important to put them where household pets cannot reach them. There are 3 main active ingredients used in rat baits. Long-Acting Anticoagulants (LAAC's), Bromethalin, and Cholecalciferol. LLAC's prevent the body from making Vitamin K which is a component needed for blood to clot. If an animal is not making Vitamin K there is a risk for them bleeding out internally. Fortunately, if an animal eats this bait and it is caught in time, prescription strength Vitamin K can be given until the animal is making it again on its own. Bromethalin is a neruo toxin and causes brain swelling. The animal will develop central nervous sign symptoms and ultimately die from seizures. Cholecalciferol is an overdose of Vitamin D which cause kidney failure.

If you suspect your pet has been exposed to something toxic, move them away from the toxin. Assess to make sure they are alert and breathing normally. Try to ascertain what was eaten and how much and then contact your veterinarian or pet poison.

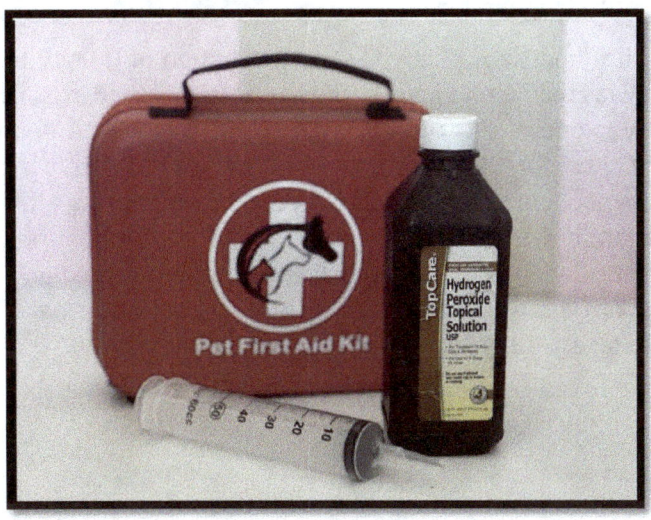

Hydrogen peroxide can induce vomiting in dogs but should never be used for cats

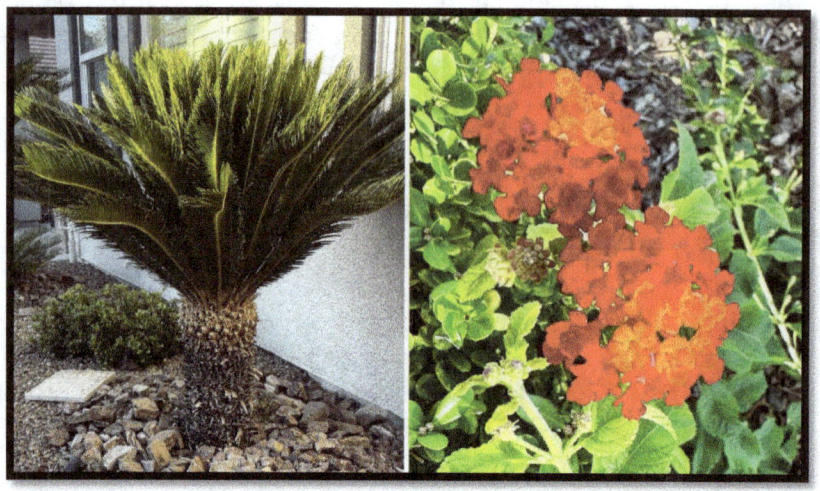

Plants such as Sago Palms (left) and Lantana (right) are commonly used in landscaping throughout the southwestern US however they are very toxic to pets

Poison Control Organizations

Pet Poison Helpline- Pet Poison Helpline is a 24-hour animal poison control service available throughout the U.S., Canada, and the Caribbean for pet owners and veterinary professionals who require assistance with treating a potentially poisoned pet. They have the ability to help every poisoned pet, with all types of poisonings, 24 hours a day. Like the ASPCA, their phone service charges a fee.

ASPCA- The American Society for the Prevention of Cruelty to Animals® (ASPCA®) was the first humane society to be established in North America and today is one of the largest in the world. The ASPCA Animal Poison Control Center (APCC) is a resource for any animal poison-related emergency, 24 hours a day, 365 days a year. There is a charge for the phone consultation, however they have a free app that can be downloaded on smartphones and tablets. It provides critical information on toxins including pictures for identification, level of toxicity, side effects and actions to take. Visit www.aspca.org for more information.

Snake Bites

Venomous snakes can reside in many areas of the US. These dangerous creatures can pose a life-threatening hazard to your pets. The Unites States has a multitude of venomous snakes in each region.

To find out what types of venomous snakes are in your area visit:

www.venombyte.com/venom/snakes/venomous_snakes_by_stat e.a sp

What do you do if a snake bites a pet?

Well, first it's worth mentioning what you do not do:

- Do not take out a pocketknife and cut Xs over the fang marks
- Do not attempt to suck venom out of the bite wounds.

Instead, you should try to identify the snake by taking note of its size, color patterns and the presence or absence of a rattle at the end of the tail. Look the pet over carefully for fang marks, noting that there may be more than one bite wound. Start your journey to the nearest animal hospital as quickly as possible while trying to keep the pet as quiet and still as possible. The more your pet moves around, the faster the venom will circulate throughout its body.

Gold standard treatment for snakebite is antivenom, IV fluids, and pain medication. Most general practices don't carry antivenom and the patient may need to be treated at an emergency center or referral center. Snake bites cause extreme swelling and are very painful. Giving antihistamines like Benadryl is not recommended as the swelling is not being caused by a histamine reaction. Steroids, NSAID's (Non-Steroidal Anti-Inflammatory Drugs) and antibiotics are also contraindicated. Very few snake bites get infected, so antibiotics are not needed. Pit Viper venom causes issues with blood being able to clot, which is why NSAID's are not recommended. Treatment should include blood work to monitor clotting profiles.

Rattlesnakes, Copperheads, and Water Moccasins (Cotton Mouths) are all pit vipers and treatment is the same regardless of species. Coral Snakes bites require a different anti-venom. If your pet is bitten by a non-venomous snake, simply wash the wound with soap and water.

Preventing Snake Bites

While out walking, controlling the dog with a leash may be your best safety device.

- Do not allow the dog to explore holes in the ground or dig under logs, flat rocks or planks.
- Stay on open paths where there is an opportunity for snakes to be visible. Keep nighttime walks to a minimum; rattlers are nocturnal most of the year.
- If you hear a rattlesnake, keep the dog at your side until you locate the snake. Then move away.
- Off-trail hiking with an unleashed dog may stir up a snake and you may be as likely a victim as the dog. If the dog seems unusually curious about something hidden in the grass, back off immediately until you know what it is.

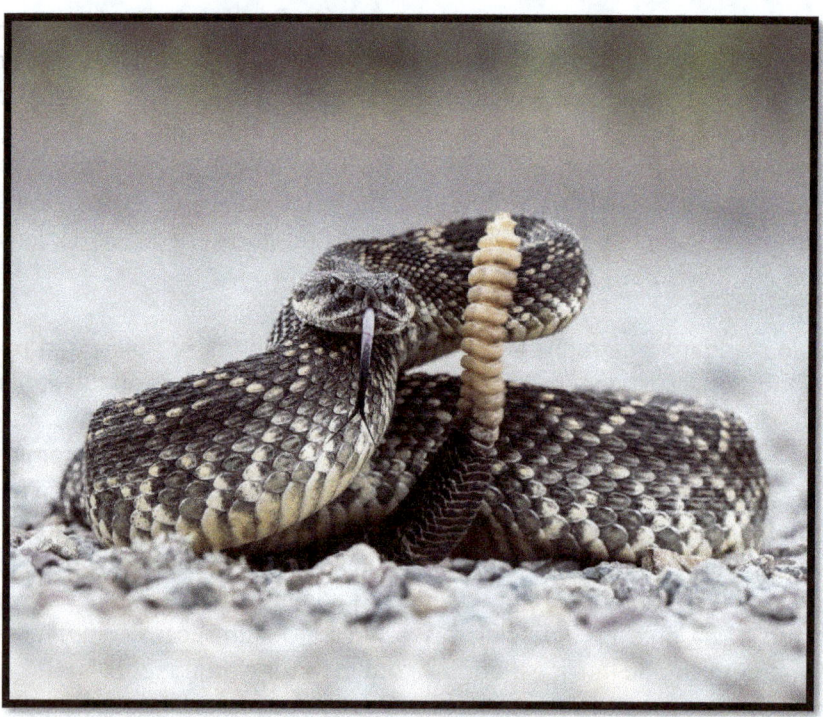

Shock

Shock is when the animal's organs do not receive enough oxygenated blood. They will begin to function slowly and then begin to die. There are many different situations that can cause shock. Some of these include excessive bleeding, hit by car, hypothermia, hyperthermia, seizures, trauma, and severe allergic reactions.

There are 3 types of shock:

Hypovolemic: This type of shock occurs when there has been a significant loss of blood or fluid due to an injury.

Cardiogenic: When the heart has failed, cardiogenic shock will occur.

Distributive: Most associated with infections, distributive shock results from problems within peripheral blood vessels and causes blood to flow away from the central circulatory system.

Signs of shock include:
- Anxiety
- Changes in the level of responsiveness
- Rapid shallow breaths
- Extreme thirst
- Extremities being cold
- Trembling, collapse
- Dilated pupils
- Gums extremely pale or showing a bluish discoloration

First aid for shock needs to be administered as quickly as possible. This is an extremely life-threatening situation for the animal. Prompt recognition of the signs, immediate initiation of first aid procedures, and safe and rapid transport to a veterinary hospital may save the animal's life.

Be prepared to provide adequate CPR if the animal goes into cardiac arrest. If the animal is bleeding from its injuries, you need to stop the bleeding. Gently immobilize the pet and prevent loss of body heat by covering the animal with one or more blankets. It is helpful to keep the animal's head lower than its heart so that blood continues to flow to the brain. Immediately transport the animal to a veterinary hospital.

Seizures

Seizures are one of the most frequently reported neurological conditions in dogs. The scientific term for seizure is "ictus". A seizure may also be called a convulsion or fit and is a temporary involuntary disturbance of normal brain function that is usually accompanied by uncontrollable muscle activity. Epilepsy is used to describe repeated episodes of seizures. With epilepsy, the seizures can be single or may occur in clusters, and they can be infrequent and unpredictable or may occur at regular intervals. Seizures are more common in dogs than cats.

There are many causes of seizures. Idiopathic epilepsy, the most common cause of seizures in the dog, is an inherited disorder, but its exact cause is unknown. Other causes include liver disease, kidney failure, brain tumors, brain trauma, or toxins. Seizures often occur at times of changing brain activity, such as during excitement or feeding, or as the dog is falling asleep or waking up. Affected dogs can appear completely normal between seizures.

Despite the dramatic and violent appearance of a seizure, seizures are not painful, although the dog may feel confusion and perhaps panic. Contrary to popular belief, dogs do not swallow their tongues during a seizure. If you put your fingers or an object into its mouth, you will not help a pet and you run a high risk of being badly bitten or of injuring the dog.

The important thing is to keep the dog from falling or hurting itself by knocking objects onto itself and it is best not to touch the animal while it is having a seizure. It is helpful to time how long the seizure lasts and report that information to the veterinarian. If the dog is on the floor or ground, there is little chance of harm occurring. Veterinary medical treatment is usually begun only after a pet has had more than one seizure a month, clusters of seizures where one seizure is immediately followed by another or grand mal seizures that are severe or prolonged in duration.

A single seizure is rarely dangerous to the dog. However, if the dog has multiple seizures within a short period of time (cluster seizures), or if a seizure continues for longer than a few minutes, the body temperature begins to rise. If hyperthermia or an elevated body temperature develops secondary to a seizure, another set of problems may have to be addressed.

Trauma/Hit by Car (HBC)

When an animal is hit by a car there is a great deal of trauma to their body that can result. It also becomes a very emotionally charged environment, especially if it is your animal. Most vehicular accidents involving animals usually involves a dog. Since the accident results in the animal being in the road it is important to safely move the animal out of the line of traffic to prevent further injury to both the pet and the rescuer. If there are any bystanders, ask them to help stop traffic and assist you if you are unable to carry the animal by yourself.

Remember that animals that are in pain and are scared can lash out by biting and/or scratching. Have your gauze muzzle handy if you need to place one on the animal or a pillowcase in the case of wrapping up a cat. If the animal is having trouble breathing, then do not place anything on its head. *Refer to the section in this book about how to safely move an injured animal.*

Observe the animal carefully to evaluate them for wounds, in particular wounds that are bleeding. Take some clean gauze from your first aid kit or a clean cloth to put pressure on the wound. If you suspect any type of head trauma, or other fractures or breaks, use caution when moving the animal. Further movement to areas of the body that sustained serious wounds can cause the injuries to become much worse. Consider putting a splint on the animal's limb to immobilize the limb during transport. Animals that go into cardiac arrest will need to have CPR initiated and likely continued until you get to a veterinary hospital. Internal injuries from such an accident may not show up until 12-72 hours after the accident. Therefore, it is so important to get the animal to a veterinarian to be evaluated even if the event seemed minor.

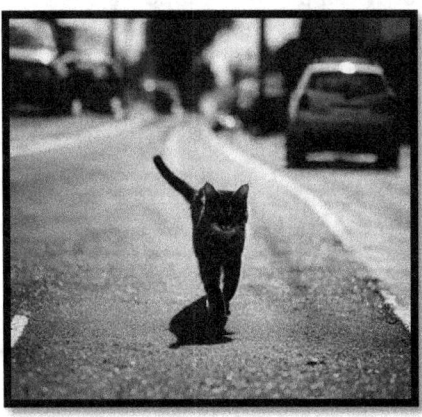

Most hit by cars happen to dogs but cats that are allowed outdoors are also at risk

Wounds and Wound Management

Wounds in animals come in different types and severity. They happen for a variety of reasons and can be considered minor to severe in nature. Most pet wounds are general and can be considered a basic first-aid situation, while other wounds are considered traumatic, and are considered an emergency. For people to understand what to do with a wound, they must first understand what kind of wound their animal has sustained. It is important to also understand the healing process of wounds, and what the treatment options are.

The first step in managing any type of wound is to stop any bleeding. It is also important to be as clean as possible to minimize infection. To stop bleeding hold a clean cloth, sterile dressing, or sanitary napkin against the wound. Keep firm pressure on the area for at least 5 minutes. If blood flow is strong it is important to get the animal to a veterinary hospital as quickly as possible, so the animal does not lose too much blood. It only takes the loss of 2 tsp. of blood per pound of body weight for an animal to go into shock. DO NOT remove the bandage until the bleeding stops or you get to a veterinarian. Removing the absorbent material too soon can disrupt the clot that is forming. Add additional material if needed. If the animal's bleeding has not stopped within 15 to 20 minutes, you must transport the animal to the veterinarian as quickly as possible.

Classifications of wounds:

- *Clean wound-* A wound made under sterile conditions where there are no organisms present in the wound and the wound is likely to heal without complications.

- *Contaminated wound-* The wound is a result of accidental injury where there are pathogenic organisms and foreign bodies in the wound.

- *Infected wound-* The wound has pathogenic organisms present and multiplying showing clinical signs of infection, where it looks yellow, oozing pus, having pain and redness.

- *Colonized wound- The* wound is a chronic one and there are a number of organisms present and very difficult to heal.

Types of Wounds

Abrasions- Abrasions occur when the superficial layers of skin are scraped, causing a minor area of inflammation, surface bleeding, and bruising. The most common cause for this can be the pet scratching or chewing at an area. The pet can also cause abrasions by jumping fences, fighting, being dragged by an automobile, or from a leash. In most cases abrasions are minor and can be treated at home, healing uneventfully. You can clean an abrasion by using antibacterial soap and warm water. Gently rinse the area removing any dirt and debris. Most abrasions are minor and can be managed by applying a triple antibiotic to the area twice a day and keeping the wound clean making sure the pet does not lick or scratch at the area. Any abrasion that has not started to heal within a few days should be taken to a veterinarian.

Lacerations- Lacerations occur when the skin is cut or torn open. Depending on what caused the laceration, the result can be a wound that has clean edges and is well-defined and only superficial in nature, or the wound can have jagged edges and be dirty, affecting several layers of the skin and into the muscle tissue. Any laceration injury that also severed any blood vessels will likely need to have the bleeding stopped first before managing the wound. Lacerations are painful so use caution when touching the animal. If you are able, rinse the wound once the bleeding has stopped to remove any dirt or debris. Due to the severity of a laceration, it is recommended to seek veterinary attention for the pet.

Bite Wounds/Puncture Wounds- Objects that pierce the skin, leaving a small hole on the surface, are considered a puncture wound. When this occurs, bacteria can enter the wound and cause an infection at a rapid rate. Cat bite wounds tend to be small puncture wounds that become infected very quickly. Dog bites can be large punctures involving deep layers of skin and muscle, or they can also appear as gashes - usually around the neck or ear of your dog. Puncture/bite wounds can be very painful, especially if your pet was picked up by the teeth of another animal and shaken. Their fur easily disguises bite wounds on dogs and cats, and they can develop into an abscess if the owner does not notice them right away. Do not be afraid to let the wound bleed unless it is gushing out or seems like a large amount of blood is being lost. Since puncture wounds, especially bite wounds, are very infectious, letting it bleed a little will help move bacteria out of the wound.

After 5 minutes, if it is still bleeding, stop the bleeding through direct pressure as described in the bleeding section above. If the bleeding stops, cleanse the wound with a safe disinfectant such as Curicyn©, Iodine or hydrogen peroxide. Animals with puncture wounds will likely need antibiotics so it is strongly suggested to seek veterinary treatment.

Supplies Needed to Administer First Aid for Wounds:

- Rolled gauze
- Non-adhesive wrap
- Porous tape
- Cotton balls
- Cotton swabs
- Bandage Scissors
- Antiseptic ie. Iodine, Chlorhex, Curicyn, etc.
- Splints
- Gauze pads
- Compression bandage
- Gloves
- Sterile water or saline
- Blood stop powder

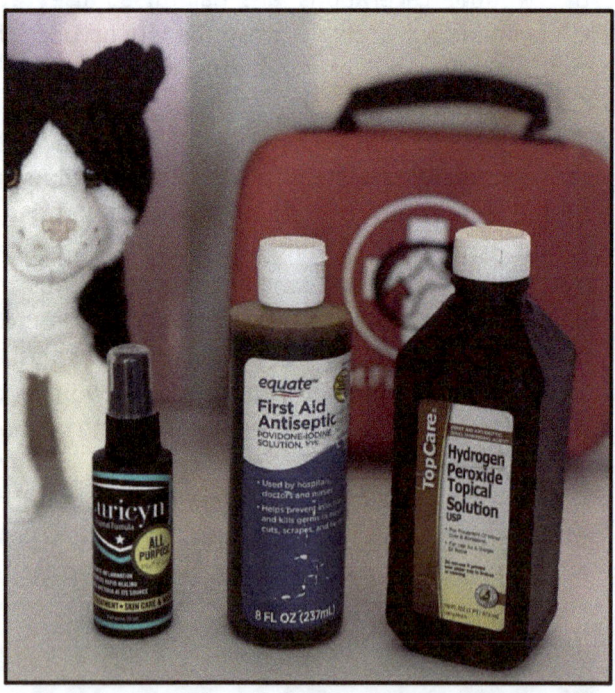

Antiseptics are a necessity to properly clean and disinfect a wound

Bandaging- A bandage is a piece of material used to support a dressing or splint, to provide protection to a wound or to restrict the movement of a part of the body. Other bandages are used without dressings, such as elastic bandages that are used to reduce swelling or provide more stringent support. These tight bandages can be used to slow blood flow to an extremity, such as when a limb is bleeding heavily. Bandages can often be improvised, as the situation demands, using clothing, blankets or other material and are placed using three layers of dressing. Only a trained individual should place a bandage on a pet. Bandages that are placed too tight or too loose can sometimes cause more damage than the injury itself.

- A *splint* is a device used for support or immobilization of a limb. It can be used in multiple situations, including temporary immobilization of potentially broken bones or damaged joints.

- *Sling-* a style of bandage used in dogs and cats that holds the foreleg or hind leg in flexion with the hip in abduction and internal rotation or holds up the abdominal area so the animal can be moved. This holds the body part up so that the animal does not put weight on it potentially damaging the injured limb further. The sling is an especially useful bandage. If a sling is applied incorrectly on a limb, blood supply to the limb can be compromised leading to serious consequences.

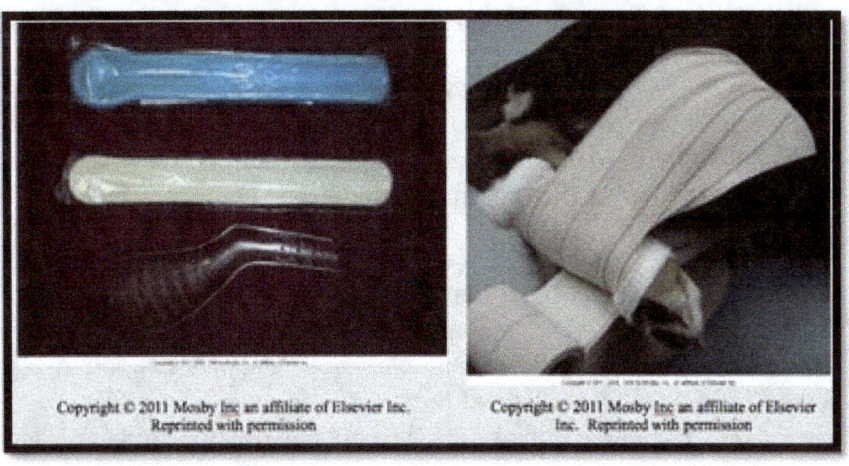

The pictures above show (left) commercial splints and (right) an Ehmer Sling

Applying a splint

Step 1- Examine the animal's wound before attempting to clean it or create a splint. Check if the wound is still actively bleeding or if the blood is mostly dry. If the wound continues to bleed profusely, you need to get the animal to a veterinary specialist as soon as possible. Put on a pair of plastic gloves and gently push aside any hair obscuring the wound. Note the size and depth of the injury. Some broken or fractured bones do not produce any external wound at all, so the lack of blood does not necessarily mean the animal's leg is not damaged. Step 2- Hold the animal still, or have a helper hold him still if someone is available to help, and gently rinse the wound with water or a light saline solution. Hold the hair around the wound aside if it is in the way. Do not move suddenly or touch the animal's injury directly, as this may frighten the pet and make them aggressive. Flush the wound with a low-concentration or non-astringent antiseptic. Absorb excess liquid remaining on the wound by dabbing it gently with a clean cloth or gauze.

Step 3- Bandage the animal's leg by wrapping the cloth strip around it multiple times. Pull it so it lays snug against the animal's leg without applying pressure to the wound. Layer the bandage by wrapping it around the injured area several times. Wind it around the skin above and below the injury as well. Seal the loose end of the bandage with medical tape to keep it in place.

Step 4- Fit the splint slowly around the animal's entire leg. For ankle injuries, the splint material should cover the paw, ankle, and knee. If the fracture is further up the leg, then the splint should contain the entire leg up to the joint with the animal's abdomen. Wrap the splint material around the leg firmly, but not tight enough to apply pressure to the wound. Tape the splint together at the top and the base. Tug gently on the splint to make sure the tape holds.

Step 5- Take the animal to a veterinarian or an animal hospital as soon as you can. A trained specialist with access to advanced equipment, including X-ray machines, can diagnose the problem and develop a solution to fix it. In many cases, the pet will need to continue to wear a splint for several days or weeks until the bone heals. The bandage will need to be replaced regularly for the wound can be cleaned, so you will need to remove and attach the splint at least once a day during the first week or two.

Applying a Sling

There are two different types of emergency slings that you can use for animals. The first one is an abdominal sling that wraps around the animal's abdomen and supports the animal as it walks. This is helpful if the animal hurts a hind leg or joint and cannot put pressure on its hind end.

You can use a blanket or towel folded up the long way, wrap it under the animal's abdomen and hold both ends of the blanket up in the air supporting the animal's body. The other type of splint is an Ehmer sling which uses a stretchy bandage material to hold one hind leg up in flexion. This protects the limb from further harm in an injury where bearing weight could lead to further damage.

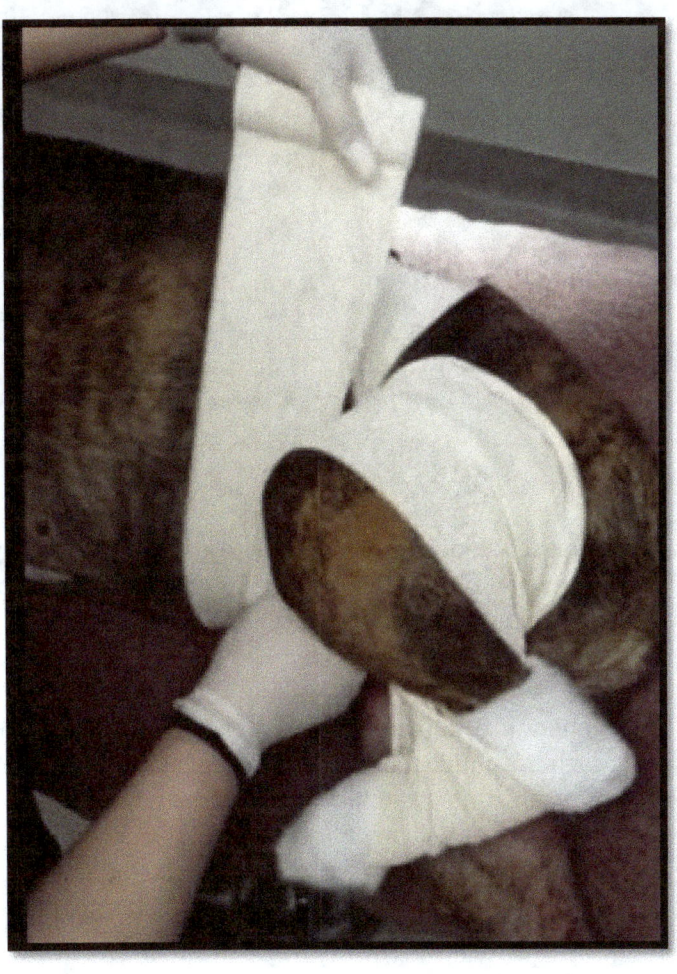

Cardiopulmonary Arrest

Cardiopulmonary arrest (CPA) occurs when normal blood circulation ceases due to the heart's inability to contract (heart failure). Like many other body systems, the respiratory and cardiovascular systems work in a coordinated fashion. Cardiac arrest can occur in dogs and cats of any age, sex, or breed. Cardiac arrest can occur due to many circumstances. From end-stage disease, to arrhythmias, to different types of cancer, cardiopulmonary arrest is an unfortunate complication of many injuries and illnesses. [4]

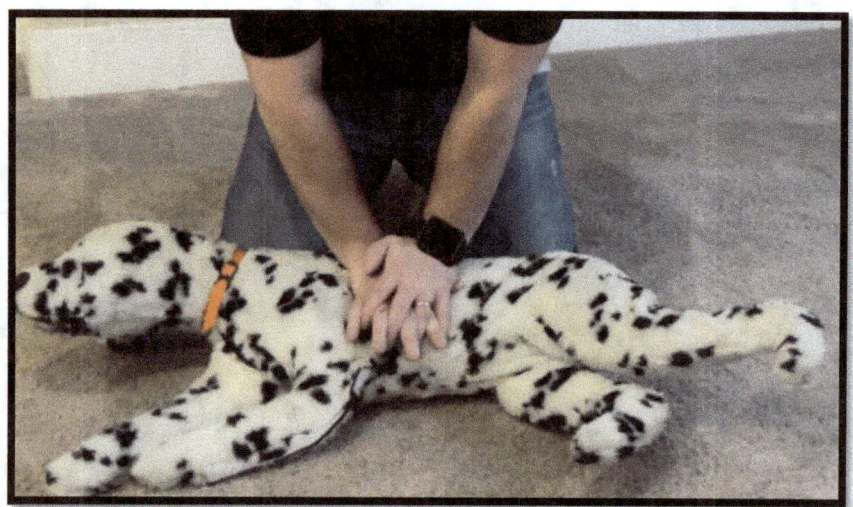

The Heart

The heart is a muscular organ about the size of a fist that pumps blood through the network of arteries and veins called the cardiovascular system. The heart pumps blood with a rhythm determined by a group of pace-making cells in the sinoatrial node.

These cells generate a current that causes contraction of the heart, traveling through the conduction system of the heart. The heart receives blood low in oxygen from systemic circulation. From here it is pumped through the lungs where it receives oxygen and gives off carbon dioxide. Oxygenated blood then returns to the heart and is pumped out to the body.

The heart has four chambers:

- The right atrium receives blood from the veins and pumps it to the right ventricle.

- The right ventricle receives blood from the right atrium and pumps it to the lungs, where it is loaded with oxygen.

- The left atrium receives oxygenated blood from the lungs and pumps it to the left ventricle.

- The left ventricle (the strongest chamber) pumps oxygen-rich blood to the rest of the body. The left ventricle's vigorous contractions create our blood pressure.

Anatomy of the Heart

Heart Anatomy. Digital image. *Www.texasheart.org*. Texas Heart Institute, n.d. Web. 13 Jan. 2017.

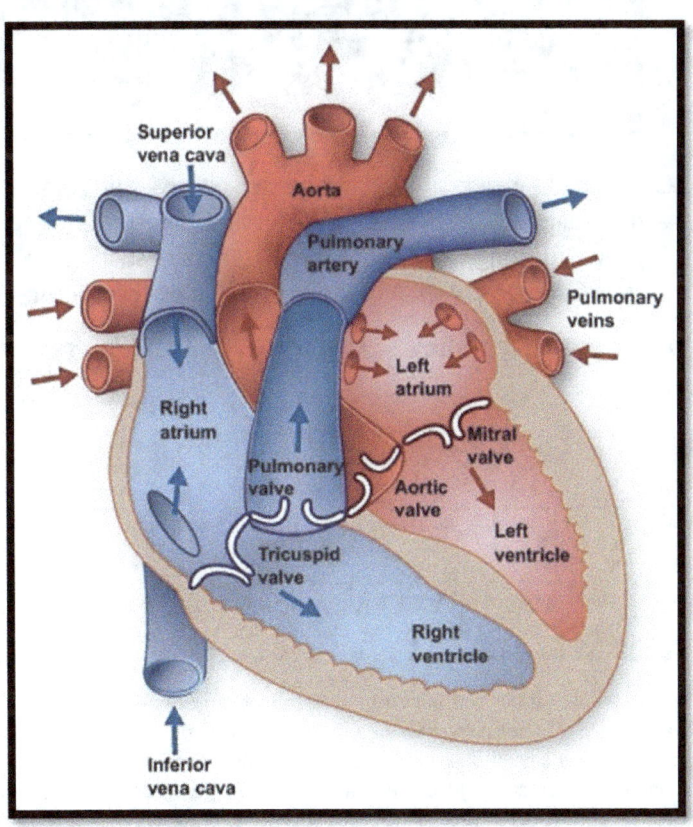

Cardiopulmonary Resuscitation

Cardiopulmonary resuscitation, commonly known as CPR, is an emergency procedure that combines chest compression with respiratory ventilation to manually preserve intact brain function until the animal reaches emergency veterinary care or the animal revives, referred to as ROSC or return to spontaneous circulation. CPR needs to begin within 10 minutes after becoming unresponsive.

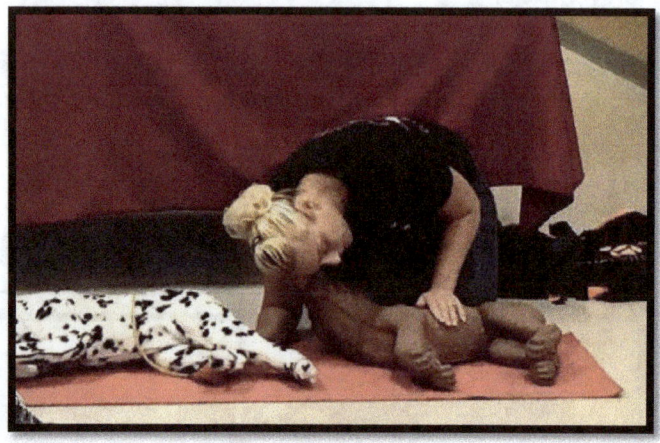

After 10 minutes, <u>irreversible</u> damage to tissues and organs begins reducing the likelihood of a successful resuscitation attempt. Injury to the patient from performing CPR is rare, however, risks such as rib fractures (1.6%), Muscle damage (14%) and Chest pain (11.7%) can occur. [3]

The following chart shows the three levels of resuscitation authorization:

Red	Do not resuscitate
Yellow	Closed chest CPR only
Green	Open chest CPR is approved by owner**

**Open chest resuscitation is usually only offered at large emergency centers or local referral centers. Some indications for open chest CPR include: Large /giant breed barrel-chested dogs, pleural specie disease, pericardial disease, patients in which closed check CPR has been unsuccessful and current abdominal surgery. Open chest resuscitation requires a large amount of aftercare including surgery to close the animal's chest. Be sure to speak with your veterinarian before choosing this option. [4]

Primary Survey

Should not take more than 15 seconds to complete

AIRWAY: Check for a clear airway. Ensure the mouth and throat are clear of any obstructions. If an obstruction is ascertained, then use the choking measures discussed earlier to dislodge the object and clear the airway.

BREATHING: Observe if the animal is breathing and if they are breathing effectively, meaning is there any extra effort taken by the animal to inhale air?

CIRCULATION: Check for a heartbeat. Palpate the femoral or other distal arterial pulse. Feel the gums, ears, and extremities to see if they are cool. See if there is any evidence of bleeding. Look for any bruising. If you have a stethoscope handy, listen to the left side of the animal's chest right behind the elbow to see if you hear any heart sounds.

Chest Compressions

There are two techniques for performing chest compressions. It has been shown that even the best-performed compressions only produce 30% of the normal stroke volume in the animal. The primary goals of chest compressions are to replace the function of the left and right ventricles, provide blood flow to the lungs, and oxygenate the tissues.

Thoracic Pump Theory- (most dogs and barrel-chested dogs) recoil of the chest between compressions causes negative pressure within the chest, drawing blood into the blood vessels and into the heart.

Cardiac Pump Theory- (cats, keel chested dogs) left and right ventricles of the heart are directly compressed between the sternum (breastbone) and the spine when compressions are done in the barrel-chested position or between the ribs on the opposite sides of the chest when in lateral recumbence (laying on their right side).

Compression Rate- Regardless of size chest, compressions should be done at a rate of 100-120 compressions per minute. Because cardiac output is the product of heart rate and stroke volume, lower compression rates result in reduced cardiac output, leading to lower survival rates. Higher compression rates also reduce cardiac output because they do not allow for full recoil of the chest, reducing the return of blood to the heart. Perform chest compressions in cycles of 2 minutes without interruption.

It takes approximately 1 minute of chest compressions for aortic blood pressure to reach a level that provides perfusion to the heart and tissues.

Compressor Position- The shoulders of the compressor should be directly above the hands. If the height of the table makes it impossible to keep the elbows locked while doing compressions, the compressor should use a stool, climb on the table with the animal or place the animal on the floor. Always lock your elbows and use your core muscles rather than your biceps or triceps. This will reduce fatigue and maintain optimal compression force. Hands should be placed one over the other, locking fingers if need be. [4]

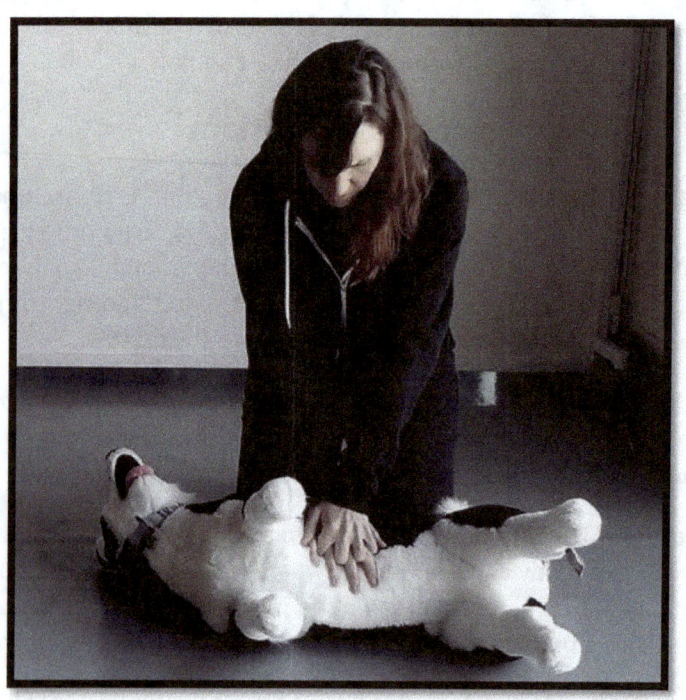

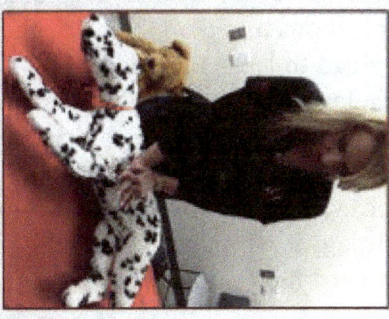

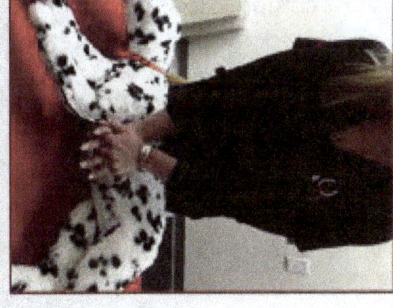

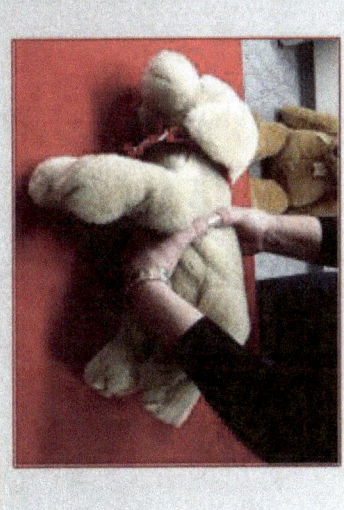

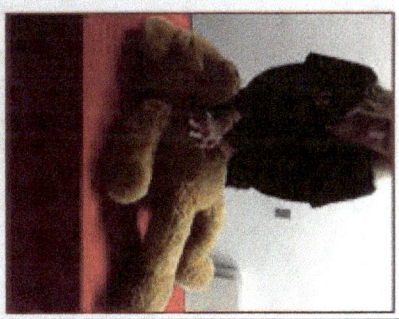

Animal Body Position for CPR

Upper left: Average Dogs- place hands over the highest point on chest

Upper middle: Keel Chested Dogs- place hands low on the check near the sternum.

Upper right: Barrel Chested Dogs- Lay animal on back and place hands on center of sternum

Lower right: Puppies, kittens, cats, small dogs- wrap hands around animal's check and compress by squeezing hands together

Note in the diagram, that dogs and cats are positioned differently for compressions based on their size and shape of their chest. Compressions in average-to-large sized dogs should be done with the hands placed over the widest portion of the animal's chest, compressions in keel chested dogs should have the hands placed directly over the heart close to the sternum, barrel chested dogs should be placed on their backs; hands are placed in the middle of the sternum for chest compressions and in cats and small dogs wrap hands around the chest and compress by squeezing thumb and fingers together. [1]

CPR Guidelines

o Chest compressions are done with the animal lying on the right side (or on back for barrel chested animals)

o Chest should be compressed at 1/2-1/3 the width of the chest

o Compression rate should be 100-120 BPM

o Make sure to allow the chest to fully recoil between compressions

o Compression ratio is 30 compressions to 2 breaths

o Perform CPR for 2 continuous minutes or 4 sets of compressions and breaths. It takes at least 1 minute of uninterrupted chest compressions to reach maximum and steady blood flow to the heart and other tissues. Pause at this time and recheck Breathing and Circulation

Airway and Breathing

The main goals of respiratory support in CPR are to ventilate the animal and increase excreted carbon dioxide produced by the tissues and provide oxygenation which transports oxygen into the blood. There are two types of pressure breaths: spontaneous and positive pressure breaths.

Spontaneous Breaths- This is when negative pressure in the chest draws air into the respiratory system on inhale. This happens during natural breathing.

Positive Pressure Breaths- This is when air is forced into the airway such as in CPR. Serious side effects of CPR can happen if the rescuer uses incorrect ventilation techniques.

Mouth-to-Snout Resuscitation

This is accomplished by pulling out the animal's tongue, closing the mouth and placing your mouth around both nostrils securely; blowing into the animal's airway watching for the chest to expand. When you feel resistance as the lungs are inflated, take your mouth off the nostrils and the lungs will deflate. Mouth to snout resuscitation breaths are not effective while the animal is being compressed, therefore you should stop compressions before breathing into the animal's airway. The reason for this is that air will flow into the esophagus and stomach rather than into the lungs when the lungs are compressed during chest compressions. [4]

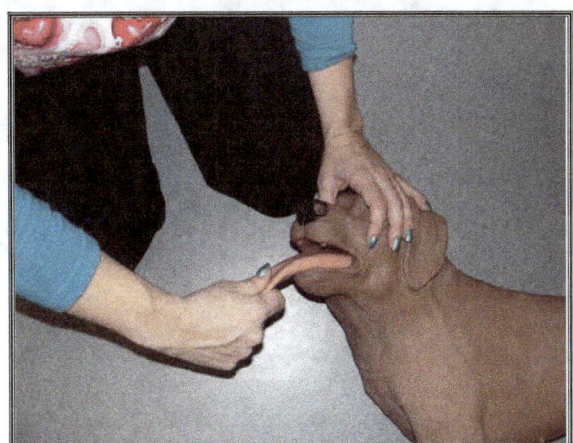

Check the animal's airway carefully for obstructions. Pull out the tongue to open the animal's airway.

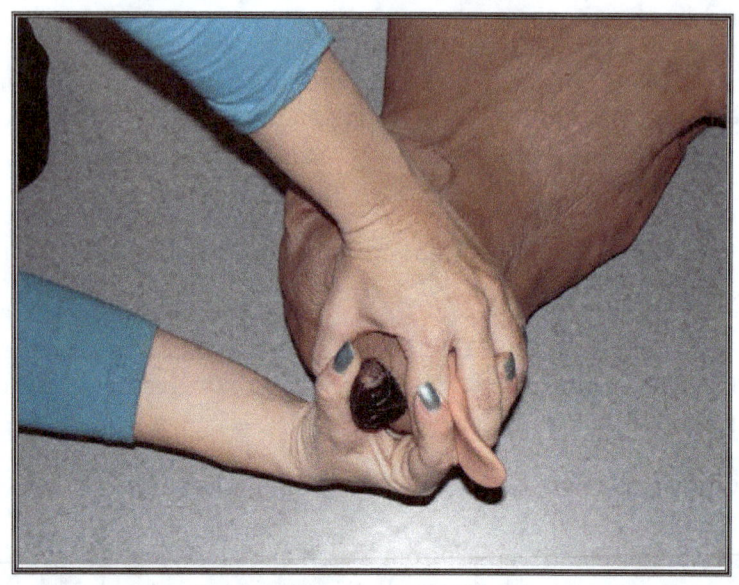

Grasp the snout, closing the mouth with your hands

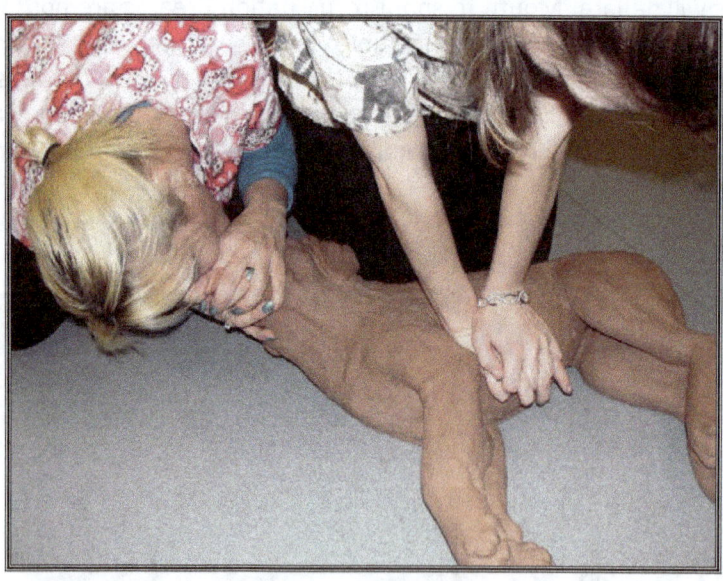

Put your mouth over the snout as pictured above, and blow into the animal's airway

Disaster Planning for Pets

What is Disaster Preparedness?

This is the process of ensuring that an owner and/or animal business has preventive measures in place so that they are in a state of readiness to contain the effects of a forecasted disastrous event to minimize loss of life, injury, and damage to property. Being prepared means that you can provide rescue, relief, rehabilitation, and other services in the aftermath of a disaster, and have the capability and resources to continue to sustain its essential functions without being overwhelmed by the demand placed on them. Preparedness for the first and immediate response is called emergency preparedness.

What is Disaster Response?

Disaster response is the second phase of the disaster management cycle. It consists of several elements such as warning/evacuation, search and rescue, providing immediate assistance, and assessingdamage.

The aim of emergency response is to provide immediate assistance to maintain life, improve health and support the morale of the affected population. Such assistance may range from providing specific but limited aid, transport from harm, temporary shelter, and food.

Knowing how to prepare for and manage an emergency that involves pets is vital. Having an appropriate plan is one of the best things you can do in terms of protecting your beloved pets in a disaster. The four phases of emergency management will give recommendations for mitigating, preparing for, responding to and recovering from all types of disasters.

What are some things that can be done at home or at the business to help prevent hazards during a disaster?

- Build and repair buildings
- Replace or cover glass windows with materials that will not shatter and injure animals and/or people
- Avoid accumulating piles of trash that can spill over and injure animals and/or people
- Store chemicals in storm proof buildings or containers and make them secure
- Do not leave construction material unsecured. High winds may cause such items to become projectile
- Drain or build levees around ponds that could flood

The priorities for disaster planning will vary to some extent with the type of animals and facility. In general terms, the greatest priorities, i.e., the most likely disasters to occur, are trailer accidents, floods, fires, power outages and contagious disease outbreaks. Some locations will have additional hazards to consider, such as high winds, landslides, and hazardous materials. Owners should consult their local emergency management office on what type of help is available and where to get it.

Many disasters also have distant effects on animals; debris many miles from a tornado touchdown and mold following a flood can be a serious problem. If you are concerned about diseases that may result from a disaster you should consult your veterinarian.

During floods, following tornadoes and earthquakes, hazardous materials can be knocked over and contaminate the environment and animals. Untrained persons should not deal with hazardous materials at all. If you are concerned about a hazardous materials release, phone 911.

Before assessing an animal, check the scene for moving traffic, power lines that are down and materials that can become explosive. These are just some examples of scenes you do not want to approach and will want to immediately call 911.

Relocation

Every pet owner should have alternative accommodations planned for their animals in the event of a disaster and contacts should be confirmed at least once per year. Become familiar with resources such as managers of fairgrounds, racetracks, etc. that may be consulted when identifying facilities that may be available. Be sure when selecting facilities to choose those that will not likely be affected by the same disasters you are planning for.

For help identifying pet-friendly lodging, you can visit these websites:
- Bringfido.com
- Dogfriendly.com
- Doginmysuitcase.com
- Pet-friendly-hotels.net
- Pets-allowed-hotels.com
- Petswelcome.com
- Tripswithpets.com

Evacuations can present unique problems. Appropriate planning is essential. Evacuations are best coordinated with neighbors, friends, local animal groups, clubs, and county extension educators. Both the destination and the method of transport need to be sorted out well in advance of any need. It is important to contact your town to find out if there are any evacuation routes predetermined in your area.

Have a plan in place as it is vital that you take your pet with you when you evacuate. Your local humane organization, agricultural extension agent, or local emergency management agency may be able to provide you with information about your community's disaster response plans. Share your evacuation plans with friends and neighbors. Post detailed instructions in several places to ensure emergency workers can see them in case you are not able to evacuate your pets yourself.

It is extremely helpful to put together a pet evacuation and disaster kit. The items can be put into any store-bought, easy-to-carry waterproof container.

Below are some recommended items for your kit:

- Food and Medicine
- 3-7 days' worth of dry and canned food
- 7 days' supply of water
- Feeding and water dish
- First aid kit
- Litter for cats
- Newspaper
- Household cleaner (not phenol based which is toxic to cats)
- Important documents as discussed in the pet first aid kit section
- Emergency contact list (see template at end of book)
- Photo of your pet preferably with you in case you get separated
- Crate or carrier
- Extra collar and leash
- ID tags on pet
- Flashlight
- Muzzle/gauze
- Toys and treats

Types of Disasters

Hurricanes- During a hurricane it is recommended that you bring your pets with you and never leave them at home. Animals left behind can get injured, become ill, starve, drown from flooding, and hamper human evacuation. Identify a place ahead of time to evacuate pets to. Be sure to identify your pets with collars and ID tags. Microchipping is also a great way to identify the pets.

Tornado- Tornados usually happen with little or no warning. Pet owners who live in tornado prone areas should make sure they have identification on all of their pets. Keep small animals such as small dogs and cats indoors. This will better protect them if a tornado strikes. It is a good idea to practice bringing your animals to a safe location before the tornado strikes. Animals can become frightened during extreme weather so practicing gathering them together, leashing dogs, etc. will help if/when the real situation happens.

Floods- Floods are an overflowing of a large amount of water beyond its normal confines, especially over what is normally dry land. You should always bring pets with you in the event of a flood. Animals left behind are likely going to drown. Identify a place ahead of time to evacuate to during a flood. Many towns and counties have flood evacuation routes already established.

Earthquake- An earthquake (also known as a quake, tremor, or temblor) is the shaking of the surface of the Earth, resulting from the sudden release of energy in the earth. Earthquakes can range in size from those that are so weak that they cannot be felt to those violent enough to toss people around and destroy whole cities. When you feel an earthquake, gather your pets, and stay inside. Seek shelter under a sturdy table away from windows and glass doors. The animals may find their own place that they feel safe inside. It is OK to let them do that. If you are outdoors go to an open area away from trees, buildings, walls and power lines. If you are driving, be sure to pull over on the side of the road and stop. Avoid parking near overpasses and power lines and do not leave the car until the shaking is over.

Home Fires- According to the American Red Cross an estimated 500,000 pets are affected by fires every year and that 1000 fires each year are started by pets. Be sure to include your pet in your family disaster plan. It is a good idea to have a pet rescue sticker on your front and back doors. You can get a sticker for free at https://secure.aspca.org/take-action/order-your-pet- safety-pack. The first thing a first responder will see on your door is that you have pet inside. For smaller animals, have a pet carrier handy enabling you can gather them and evacuate quickly. Make sure your pet is wearing identification and/or microchipped.

Wildfires- A wildfire is a fire that is out of control. It needs to be put out or suppressed. Wildfires may be caused by lightning, volcanic activity, arson, or human carelessness with campfires, cigarettes, fireworks, or machinery. It is important to have an evacuation plan in areas that are prone to wildfires. You need to be able to take your animals with you or if you are not home, identify neighbors that can help get your animals to safety. As with all disasters, make sure your pets are identified.

Volunteering to Help During a Disaster

Volunteer opportunities vary based on many factors including type of disaster, organization in charge, etc. People interested in volunteering on an animal rescue team should contact their local emergency response service, humane society, or other animal rescue agency. Many of these organizations require volunteers to apply to work with the organization and for the volunteer to be listed as a contact in case of an emergency. Your talents may be utilized as an animal care giver, rescuer that goes out and collects animals, veterinary care and more. Animal rescue volunteers often say that their experience helping animals in a disaster changed their lives. They cherish the opportunity to help animals and learned important skills as part of the efforts.

After the Disaster

Be sure to survey the area inside and outside of your home, barn, kennels, etc. Look for sharp objects, dangerous materials, contaminated water, downed power lines or other hazards. If you were separated from your animals, make sure to inspect them for harm. If you notice any signs of injury or illness, make sure to take them to a veterinarian right away. Release your pets inside only when you get home. There may be dangerous wildlife and debris outside. If allowed outside they could get hurt. Allow uninterrupted rest so that animals can recover from the trauma of the disaster. The disruption of routine activity can be a problem, so try to keep animals quiet.

If your animals are missing then immediately check all shelters, animal control stations, and the local humane society or veterinary medical response team to see if they have your animal in custody. Post waterproof lost animal notices and notify local law enforcement. Having your animal microchipped is a particularly good idea so that it is easier to locate them after a disaster.

Quick References

Careers Working with Animals

For those who have a passion for animals and a desire to make their lives better. Working with animals isn't just a job; it's a calling that combines compassion, dedication, and a deep understanding of the animal kingdom. Whether it's nurturing the health and well-being of pets as a veterinary professional, training dogs to assist people with disabilities, or caring for exotic animals in a zoo, each career path offers its unique rewards and challenges. Beyond the joy of working with animals, these careers also play a crucial role in conservation, public education, and enhancing the bond between humans and animals.

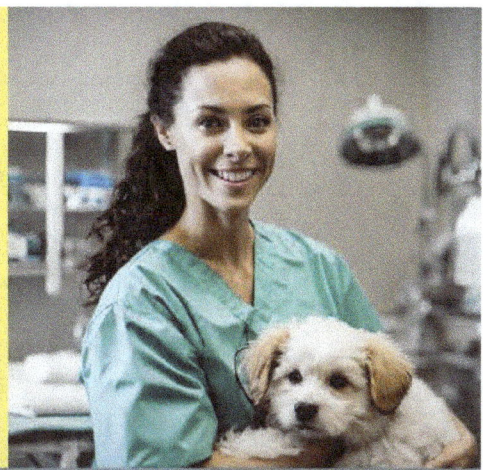

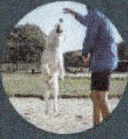

Animal Trainer

Animal trainers work with animals to teach them tricks and behaviors. Animal trainers need to be patient, understand how animals think and feel, and know a lot about the particular animal they are working with. It's a cool job if you love animals and enjoy teaching and working with them!

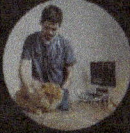

Veterinary Staff

Working in a veterinary hospital is a bit like working in a hospital for humans, but your patients are animals. This career can be really interesting and rewarding, especially if you love animals. There are different roles in a veterinary hospital including veterinarian, veterinary nurse technician or receptionist to name a few.

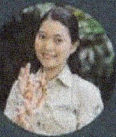

Zookeeper

A career as a zookeeper is like being a caretaker and guardian for animals that live in a zoo. If you love animals and are interested in their well-being, this could be a great job for you. As a zookeeper, your main role is to look after the animals. This includes a lot of different tasks, such as feeding, cleaning habitats and educating visitors.

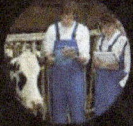

Farmer/Agriculture

Working with animals in agriculture means you're involved in the care and management of animals that are raised for products like milk, meat, eggs, and wool. This career is a blend of outdoor work, animal care, and understanding how a farm operates.

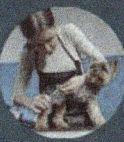

Pet Groomer

Pet groomers bathe, brush, and trim the hair of pets. They may also provide other services such as nail trimming and ear cleaning.

Summary

These are just a few of the many different jobs that involve working with animals. If you love animals, there are many opportunities to find a career that allows you to work with them.

Pain Scale for Dogs and Cats (fig. b1)

Feline Scale

Score	Description
0	No pain, no overt signs of discomfort and no resentment to firm pressure
1	Some pain, no overt signs of discomfort but resentment to firm pressure
2	Moderate pain, some overt signs of discomfort which are made worse by
3	Severe pain, obvious signs of persistent discomfort which are made worse

Canine Scale

Score	Criteria
Vocalization	
0	No vocalization
1	Vocalizing responds to calm voice and stroking
2	Vocalizing does not respond to calm voice and stroking
Movement	
0	None
1	Frequent position changes
2	Thrashing
Agitation	
0	Asleep or calm
1	Mild agitation
2	Moderate agitation
3	Severe agitation

Medical Abbreviations

ABC- Airway, Breathing, Circulation

ABN- Abnormal

ALS- Advanced Life Support

BLS- Basic Life Support

BPM- Beats per Minute

BS- Breath Sounds

CCU- Critical Care Unit

CHD- Chronic Heart Disease

CHF- Congestive Heart Failure

CO- Cardiac Output

COAD- Chronic Obstructive Lung Disease

CPA- Cardiopulmonary arrest

CPR- Cardiopulmonary resuscitation

CRT- Capillary Refill Time

CV- Cardiovascular

D/C- Discharge

DNR- Do Not Resuscitate

ECG/EKG- Electrocardiogram

FB- Foreign Body

Hx- History

HR- Heart Rate

ICU- Intensive Care Unit

INH- Inhaled

IV- Intravenous

IVF- Intravenous Fluids

Kg- Kilogram

Lb- Pounds

LOS- Loss of Consciousness

LV- Left Ventricle

O2- Oxygen

P- Pulse

Temperature

TPR- Temperature, Pulse, Respiration

Tx- Treatment

VS- Vital Signs

R- Respiration

ROSC- Return of spontaneous circulation

RR- Respiratory Rate

Glossary

Acute: sudden, intense flare up.

Airway: the path that air follows to get into and out of the lungs.

Analgesia: an unpleasant sensation that can range from mild localized discomfort to agony, pain.

Anemia: chronically low hematocrit.

Anterior: word used to describe the front surface of something.

Anti-: prefix generally meaning "against, opposite or opposing, and contrary."

Antibiotic: a drug used to treat bacterial infections.

Arrhythmia: when the beat of the heart is no longer originating from the sinus node.

Aspirate: accidental inhaling of a substance or fluid.

Blood pressure: the pressure of the blood within the arteries.

Bradycardia: also known as Brady arrhythmia, is a slow heart rate.

Bradypnea: or bradypnoea is abnormally slow breathing.

Breathing: the process of respiration, during which air is inhaled into the lungs .

Capillary Refill: the refilling of blood back into tissues.

Cardiac: having to do with the heart.

Cardiomyopathy: a disorder of the heart muscle that can be fatal.

Cardiopulmonary: having to do with both the heart and lungs.

Cardiopulmonary resuscitation: a life-saving emergency procedure that involves breathing into a victim's airway and compression their chest to deliver oxygen to the vital organs.

Critical care: a branch of medicine concerned with the diagnosis and management of life-threatening conditions requiring sophisticated organ support and invasive monitoring.

Cyanotic: when a patient's mucous membranes are bluish in color from an inadequate supply of oxygen to the blood.

Diastolic: pressure during relaxation and dilation of the heart.

Distal Pulse: the pulse farthest from the heart.

Dyspnea: difficulty breathing.

Edema: excessive accumulation of fluid.

Embolus: a blood clot.

Emergency code: a series of color references that medical facilities use to indicate the severity of a case.

Endocarditis: inflammation of the cardiac tissue.

FEMA: the Federal Emergency Management Agency, a federal agency that coordinates the response to disasters in the U.S.

Flush: a redness of the skin, typically over the cheeks or neck.

Heart: the muscle that pumps blood received from veins into arteries throughout the body.

Hypoglycemia: low blood sugar (glucose).

Hyperthermia: abnormally high body temperature.

Hyperventilation: (also called over-breathing) occurs when the rate and quantity of alveolar ventilation of carbon dioxide exceeds the body's production of carbon dioxide.

Hypervolemia: or fluid overload, is the medical condition where there is too much fluid in the blood.

Hypothermia: abnormally low body temperature.

Hypovolemia: or oligemia, (also hypovolemia or oligaemia) is a state of decreased blood volume; more specifically, decrease in volume of blood plasma.

Hypoxia: a severe deficiency of oxygen in the blood and tissues.

Lateral recumbency: a restraint where the animal is lying on its side.

Lethal: to be deadly.

Lethargy: lack of energy.

Mucous membranes: the layer of cells that line the tubular organs of the body.

Normal Sinus Rhythm: a normal heart rate.

Palpation: refers to the use of touch and feel in the process of examining a patient.

Pericardium: the sac that envelops the heart.

Pleura: the lining around the lungs.

Pulmonary Edema: fluid in the lungs.

Pulse: a pulsating artery that gives evidence that the heart is beating. Can be used to obtain a heart rate.

Poison: any substance that can cause severe organ damage or death if ingested, inhaled or contact with skin.

Pulse: the rhythmic dilation of an artery that results from beating of the heart.

Respiratory system: a biological system consisting of specific organs and structures used for the process of respiration in an organism.

Respirations: breaths or the act of breathing.

Resuscitation: The procedure of breathing into a victim during CPR, to deliver oxygen to the lungs.

ROSC: return of spontaneous circulation.

Sepsis: a life-threatening condition that arises when the body's response to infection injures its own tissues and organs.

Spinal cord: the major column of nerve tissue that is connected to the brain.

Spinal cord injury: trauma or damage to the spinal cord, the major column of nerve tissue.

Shock: inadequate circulating blood flow such that oxygen delivery is insufficient to meet cellular energy and substrate needs.

Stethoscope: an instrument used to magnify sounds produced within the body in order to determine health or diagnose a disease.

Systolic: pressure during the contraction of the heart.

Tachycardia: abnormally fast heart rate.

Tachypnea: or tachypnea, is abnormally rapid breathing.

Thermometer: a device used to measure temperature.

Topical: pertaining to a particular surface area.

Trauma: a physical or emotional injury.

Triage: the process of placing patients coming to an emergency department into different categories. This is done to decide the order in which patients will be seen. Those with life threatening or very serious conditions will receive treatment first.

Unconscious: interruption of awareness of oneself and one's surroundings.

Urinary: having to do with the function or anatomy of the kidneys, ureters, bladder.

Urinary tract: the organs of the body that produce, store, and discharge urine.

Vomit: matter from the stomach that has come up into and may be ejected beyond the mouth.

References

1. Becker, M. (2022, September 21). Reading cat and dog body language. Vetstreet. Retrieved January 15, 2023, from https://www.vetstreet.com/our-pet-experts/body-language-the-difference-between-cats-and-dogs

2. "ACVECC RECOVER Web Site." *ACVECC RECOVER Web Site*. N.p., n.d. Web. 25 Jan. 2017.

3. Bassert, Joanna M., Dennis M. McCurnin, and Dennis M. McCurnin. *McCurnin's clinical textbook for veterinary technicians*. St. Louis, MO: Elsevier Saunders, 2010. Print.

4. Boller, Manuel, and Daniel J. Fletcher. "RECOVER evidence and knowledge gap analysis on veterinary CPR. Part 1: Evidence analysis and consensus process: collaborative path toward small animal CPR guidelines." *Journal of Veterinary Emergency and Critical Care* 22.S1 (2012): n. pag. Web.

5. Fletcher, Daniel J., PhD, DVM, DACVECC, and Elizabeth Rozanski, DVM, DACVIM, DACVEC. "Veterinary Medicine." *ECornell*. Cornell University, n.d. Web. 25 Jan. 2017.

6. Hall, John (2011). Guyton and Hall textbook of medical physiology (12th ed.). Philadelphia, Pa.: Saunders/Elsevier. ISBN 978-1-4160-4574-8

7. Kahn, Cynthia M. *The Merck veterinary manual*. Whitehouse Station, NJ: Merck & Co., 2005. Print.

8. Silverstein, Deborah C., and Kate Hopper. *Small animal critical care medicine*. St. Louis, MO: Saunders/Elsevier, 2009. Print.

9. Sirios, Margi, EDd. *Principles and Practice of Veterinary Technology Elsevier Ebook on Vitalsource*. 4th ed. N.p.: Mosby Inc, 2016. Print.

10. "The Fluid Resuscitation Plan - Emergency Medicine and Critical Care." *Veterinary Manual*. N.p., n.d. Web. 25 Jan. 2017.

11. Tighe, Monica M., and Marg Brown. *Mosby's comprehensive review for veterinary technicians*. St. Louis, MO: Mosby Elsevier, 2008. Print.